a Tonics

"Because I love tea and tonics, I founded the Queen's Tea, a gathering for heart-centered businesswomen. *Chakra Tonics* beautifully pairs chakra lessons with delicious and soothing drinks that satisfy the soul, [it's] the perfect book to complement women who are redefining what it means to be spiritual and successful."

—JESSICA HADARI, founder of the Feminine Frequency Festival and the Spiritual Women Leaders Network

"What I love about *Chakra Tonics* is that your health and healing are being supported by creating fun and delicious tonics. I often feel like I am preparing drinks and treats for a party, but instead I am whipping up elixirs that balance the pH levels in my blood along with chakra energy systems. My favorite section that I use as a simple guide is the brief explanation of acid vs alkaline foods. Elise's recipes and information are a great way to have a profound healing conversation with your body, mind, and spirit."

—SAEEDA HAFIZ, author of *The Healing: One Woman's Journey from Poverty* to Inner Riches

"*Chakra Tonics* is a rejuvenating exploration of how earth and yoga nourish and awaken all aspects of our embodied vitality."

—SHIVA REA, American yogini and founder of Prana Vinyasa Yoga

"*Chakra Tonics* gives a clear understanding of the connection between mind, body, and spirit. I often teach mindfulness sessions that include the ancient Vedic concept of the chakras. Collins's book provides readers with an understanding of thousands of years of Vedic wisdom along with recipes for delicious, vital elixirs that support a holistic lifestyle. Each chapter of this volume is scholarly, engaging, and practical."

—MURALI NAIR, PhD, adjunct professor of social work at Columbia University and coauthor of *Healing Across Cultures and the Good Life: An Approach to Holistic Health*

"Elise creates a wonderful, refreshing mix with her wisdom about how to support your chakras with specific tonics, remedies, and recipes. She weaves in different yogic practices, adding a depth to explore the journey of the chakras with the gifts they offer us. With a sense of whimsy, Elise brings humor and love in this practical guide to increase your overall health, including your chakras."

—JUDITH E. PENTZ, MD, author of *Cleanse Your Body, Reveal Your Soul: Sustainable Wellbeing Through the Ancient Therapy of Panchakarma Therapy*

CHAKRA TONICS

CHAKRA TONICS

Essential Elixirs for the Mind, Body, and Spirit

Elise Marie Collins

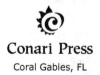

Conari Press

Coral Gables, FL

For permission requests, please contact the publisher at:
Mango Publishing Group
2850 S Douglas Road, 4th Floor
Coral Gables, FL 33134 USA
info@mango.bz

For special orders, quantity sales, course adoptions and corporate sales, please
email the publisher at sales@mango.bz. For trade and wholesale sales, please
contact Ingram Publisher Services at customer.service@ingramcontent.com or
+1.800.509.4887.

Chakra Tonics: Essential Elixirs for the Mind, Body, and Spirit

Library of Congress Cataloging-in-Publication number: 2022935522.
ISBN: (p) 978-1-64250-423-1 (e) 978-1-64250-424-8
BISAC: HEA030000, HEALTH & FITNESS / Homeopathy

Printed in the United States of America

contents

note to readers

This book is not meant to treat, diagnose, or prescribe. The information contained herein is in no way to be considered as a substitute for your own inner guidance. For any medical condition, physical condition, or symptoms, always consult with a qualified physician or appropriate health care professional. Neither the author nor the publisher accepts any responsibility for your health or how you choose to use the recipes in this book.

foreword

"Yoga" is a word from ancient Sanskrit meaning "to unite." It's not just about physical union, but also spiritual and mental wellbeing. When we separate our yoga practice into various buckets, we can miss the connection between the mental, physical, and energetic aspects of the practice. The first step in uniting the seemingly separate parts of our lives begins with understanding the connection between the energetic and the physical—always seeking ways for more integration wherever possible! *Chakra Tonics* is a rare guidebook for this reason.

Elise Collins does a masterful job joining powerful juices and tonics with the ancient energy wisdom of the chakras. The results are powerful. There is no separation between the subtle body and the gross anatomy—if you're able to heal one, you're able to heal the other. Rarely do we find a book that addresses this holistic connection in such a practical way. If you use the tonics listed in *Chakra Tonics*, you will feel more energy, mental clarity, and a greater sense of wellness.

I feel like I am part of something bigger every time I come to practice and teach yoga at Grace Cathedral. The sounds and smells all bring me back to my spiritual roots in this space where there is stillness and calm before we start our session together on the multicolored mats that cover the stone floor. There are many reasons people come to my class every week. Some just want an opportunity for self-care and reflection, while others hope that by practicing yoga, they can become more mindful of their daily lives or find peace with the world around them. We all have different goals when we show up at Grace Cathedral on Tuesday nights, but all of us find what we need in this weekly ritual.

Like the experience we share practicing yoga at Grace Cathedral, this new edition of *Chakra Tonics* includes chakra rituals that help the reader connect with their individual energy centers and find deeper connection in life. In the twenty-first century we are called upon to rethink many traditions from the past. Elise brings us timeless wisdom through simple yet powerful rituals and tonics, so you can create your own sacred experience and put these practices into practice!

—Darren Main, yoga teacher and author of *Yoga and the Path of the Urban Mystic*

introduction

The body springs from a web of energy which dances through every cell; what occurs in one portion of our physical, emotional, mental and spiritual beings is likely to have an impact on every other portion, to some degree. An understanding of this energy is useful in being able to affect the changes we want to make in our lives, including dietary transitions.

—AMADEA MORNINGSTAR, *The Ayurvedic Cookbook*

bEFORE SCIENCE came to dominate medicine, the spiritual and the metaphysical were a part of almost every culture's therapeutic practice. People knew that all living things had energetic consciousness, as did the food and drink derived from them. Fruits, vegetables, and herbs were seen as gifts from the divine that contained universal life-force energy. Sages and ordinary people, therefore, turned to the natural world to find cures not only for the body but also for the soul.

These traditional cultures often used liquids for medicinal purposes, as they were easy for the body to digest and absorb. Shamans and practitioners of Chinese medicine, *jamu*, and Ayurveda used tonics and teas in healing and religious rituals, as well as in daily life. Clearly, people understood early on the vital importance of fluids.

Today, science tells us that our bodies consist of approximately 70 percent liquid in the form of water, our blood 94 percent and our brain 90 percent. Moreover, water is an essential element of all life on Earth, covering nearly three quarters of the planet. The water element is often taken for granted, yet it is crucial to every function of our body. We can live without eating for up to a month, but without drinking we die within days. Since our bodies depend on liquids, what we imbibe greatly affects our physical and emotional health—and also our spiritual well-being. Fluids, the first nourishment we receive as babies, naturally bridge the gap between the ethereal and physical planes.

Many popular drinks consumed in Western culture are depleted of vitality. Coffee, alcohol, sodas, some processed juices, and even some types of filtered water are lifeless as well as detrimental to the physical health of the body. In the scientific approach to health, drinks are not evaluated in terms of *chi*, or universal life force. Instead, it is the amount of calories, carbohydrates, protein, vitamins, and minerals they contain that matters. When examined from a mystical point of view, on the other hand, beverages are found to be either potent vehicles of life-affirming power or transporters of soul-deadening energies. Both approaches to the question are of value. Indeed, properly applied, science can indicate health-giving properties of food and drink, as well as validate the life-enhancing abilities of many ancient practices. *Chakra Tonics* utilizes scientific research and ancient wisdom to create delicious vital elixirs for the modern body and soul.

In the Vedic tradition, we believe that we are all souls attempting to have a human experience. The chakras, which are energy portals located within the body (or in close proximity to the body) through which we process universal life-force energy. They are our link to divine origins, constantly translating the immense and immeasurable properties of the soul into our human experience. There are seven main chakras located along the spine, as well as other minor chakras located throughout the body and several out of body chakras as well. Each recipe in this book combines ingredients that relate to and focus on the functioning of a specific chakra.

Chakra tonics are healing elixirs that benefit the physical body and assist in raising the vibrational quality of life. Chakra tonics contain powerful superfoods, herbs, minerals, and pH-balanced liquids designed to affect the body's foundational energy system, the chakras. Each recipe possesses many healthful and balancing qualities and is intended to affect a certain chakra or mind-body vortex, while at the same time affecting the entire interrelated energetic body.

Many of the chakra tonics in this book are alkalizing, oxygen rich, and full of universal life-force energy. The ancient Indian sages noted the subtle influence of foods and drinks on the emotions and the spirit. Science would agree that our bodies are electrochemical laboratories in which the charge, or acid and alkaline balance, of the fluids we drink makes a tremendous difference in conducting energy through our cells, eventually influencing overall physical and psychological health.

Scientifically speaking, one of the reasons that cola, coffee, and alcohol are so detrimental to our systems is that they are acidic. The body tolerates and sometimes benefits in some cases from the consumption of acidic food and drinks; however, they must be balanced with alkaline foods and drinks. Spiritually, most processed drinks are acidic and block universal life force and leave a residue of unconsciousness that can hinder higher awareness

Many people are coming to understand that their connection to a higher power beyond the physical is intrinsic to emotional and physical health. In fact, Dr. Theodore Baroody, author of *Alkalize or Die*, says the single most alkalizing thing we can do for our body is to feel the power of the divine or "holy spirit." The Chakra tonics in this book for the most part are incredibly alkalizing and life affirming. Acid foods, drinks, and emotions must be balanced with disproportionate amounts of alkaline foods, drinks, and emotions; fresh juice; love; and herbal tea.

We are at a crucial turning point in our collective spiritual evolution. Degenerative diseases, which thrive in hyperacidic conditions brought on by stress and a Western diet, are reaching epidemic proportions. The vibration on the planet is accelerating. Now more than ever, the challenge of slowing down, taking time for a cup of tea or vital, fresh juice, is essential to those of us seeking peace and clarity or who wish to follow a more spiritual path. Instead of reaching for a prepackaged bottled tea or can of juice, take the time to prepare fresh homemade chakra tonics, which will nourish, replenish, and enthuse body and soul. Change the habitual beverages that you imbibe for the better and you will impart dramatic and extensive changes in your health, mentally, spiritually, and physically.

acid/alkaline balance

Understanding your body's pH is important in assessing the health of your fluid system, which has more water than anything else. Water's molecular structure, made up of hydrogen and oxygen (H_2O), can be ionized or separated into one positive hydrogen molecule, $H+$, and one negative hydroxyl ion, or $OH-$. Potential for hydrogen, or pH, measures the proportion of $OH-$ and $H+$ ions in any solution.

The pH scale ranges between one and fourteen. When there is an equal proportion of $OH-$ and $H+$, the pH is neutral, with a pH of seven. Most body tissues operate in a narrow range with a pH of about 7.4. When the body becomes either too alkaline, above 7.5, or too acidic, below 7.3, it can be dangerous to one's health. As the pH level goes up, the relative alkalinity or acidity increases exponentially. An 8.1 pH is ten times more alkaline than an eight pH, and a four pH ten times more acidic than a 4.1. A pH of 6.5 is 100 times more acidic than 7.5.

Even more alarming is the fact that to neutralize drinking one twelve-ounce soda with a pH of 2.5, you need to drink thirty-two glasses of alkaline water. Excess acidity is far more common today because many people are taxing their body with highly acidic foods, drinks, and stressors. In general, Americans tend to consume acidic foods and drinks, like fast food, processed food, meat, poultry, carbonated sodas, alcoholic beverages, and coffee. In addition, stress and stressful emotions—anger, fear, jealousy, overwork— are all acidic to our system.

Meditation, love, and compassion, are alkalizing. So are most herbal teas, fresh fruit and vegetable juices, smoothies, and the chakra tonics in this book. They will assist you in offsetting the acidity in your body. For further information, read Alkalize or Die by Dr. Theodore Baroody.

why chakra tonics now?

First mentioned in Vedic texts around 700 BC, the chakras are seven psychoenergetic circular centers that run from the base of the spine to the top of the head. Chakras don't exist as part of human physiology but are centers of meditative focus associated with elements (earth, water, fire, air, space) and seven areas of the body:

1. root, found at the tailbone
2. sacral, below navel
3. solar plexus, below rib cage
4. heart, chest
5. throat, neck
6. third eye, between eyebrows
7. crown, crown of head

The chakras are associated not only with areas of the body and nearby organs but also with the senses. The chakras have been compared to models of human development, similar to Maslov's hierarchy of needs and Erik Erikson's stages of psychosocial development, because they conceptualize stages of personal evolution and maturation. Sometimes we miss out on developing different parts of our inner or outer identities. In the quest for self-mastery, we can use the chakras as a template for development, because it's never too late to mature and grow spiritually, psychologically, and emotionally. We may also need to heal physical ailments, understanding the chakras can support all layers of the healing process, mentally, emotionally, and spiritually.

For example, the sacral, or Svadhisthana center, located in the lower back at the sacrum, includes our feeling of safety or belonging, sensuality, and gender identity. As six-month-old infants, we develop the sacral center as we attach to our parents, and it continues to develop as we learn about the world through our senses, go through puberty, reach sexual maturity, and continue to develop our gender identities as adults.

The third chakra, or Manipura center, is at the solar plexus and conducts physical and subtle energy through the body. It governs physical digestion and emotional and mental assimilation of knowledge. We develop the belly center as a toddler seeking autonomy, as a teenager breaking free from parental authority, and throughout life when solidifying personal power.

This book goes into more depth about the chakras, including how they relate to stages of development and how to use them as tools for psychological and spiritual growth. Using the chakras as a guide, you can more easily evolve emotionally, spiritually, and mentally. Chakras incorporate the concept that we engage in life through interwoven layers of existence, through mind, body, and spirit. For example, if you smell a rose, it affects the physical biology of your olfactory system, sparks a memory of receiving roses as a gift from your significant other, and alters the subtle quality of your heart.

The chakras can help you conceptualize healing your body holistically, instead of only suppressing symptoms. If you have a stomach ulcer, you must get physical treatment and then you can address the underlying psychological issues related to the belly center to regain your health. In *The Heart Speaks: A Cardiologist Reveals the Secret Language of Healing,* Mimi Guarneri writes about her experience as a cardiologist. With no training or understanding of the chakras, she offers a profound description of how the heart chakra functions. Dr. Guarneri was a pioneer in treating heart patients with stents. She found, however, that while she could successfully unblock her patient's arteries, she usually provided only a temporary fix. Many of Guarneri's patients returned, needing another stent or procedure, often soon after the original operation. Guarneri discovered how she could support patients healing from heart disease by helping them address underlying issues, or what could be described as heart chakra imbalances or blocks, such as loneliness, lack of self-love, or a need for forgiveness toward oneself or others. When she gave heart opening "prescriptions," such as volunteering for an organization, getting a dog, making new friends, or developing a daily gratitude practice, her patients were often able to recover and heal from chronic heart conditions.

The chakras provide a path to develop one's higher self or a "best version" of you. We are human, yet we all have a divine imprint, as a story of Krishna explains. When Krishna was a toddler, his brother and other children climbed up trees to pick fruit. Because he was so small and could not get to the delicious fruit, Krishna began to eat mud in frustration. The other children tattled on him to his mother, Yashoda. In anger, Yahoda asked him if he had eaten mud, and Krishna, being a human child, denied it. Yashoda asked him to open his mouth so she could look for mud. As Krishna opened his mouth, Yashoda became dizzy and disoriented. Inside her son's mouth she saw the sun, stars, mountains, galaxies, planets, all people, plants, and animals. Nothing was left out, even the space between everything was there. Just as Krishna is human and divine, we are divine and human and have aspects of all of creation inside us.

The chakras give us a map to uncover what my favorite yoga teacher, Judith Hansen Lasater, calls our inherent goodness or inner divinity. You don't need to be religious or have a spiritual practice to unite with your inner goodness. The chakras offer a model to understand how unseen forces of consciousness flow through the universe.

You can use the chakras as tools to grow psychologically, especially in ways where you may be deficient or where you are not living to your potential. Consider what you need to balance in your life rather than follow a prescriptive, one-size-fits-all health plan. The chakras are based on an elemental system of balance: when you make a deposit in one element, you will need to equalize it with its opposite or balancing element. The root center element is the earth; the sacral center, the element of water; the belly center, the element of fire; the heart center, the element of air; and the throat center is the element of space, or ether.

Think about when you travel by plane. You build up a lot of air, so you will need more attention to water and earth elements afterward to balance the excess air element. Otherwise, you may become depleted and risk exhaustion or possible illness. A buildup of the air element happens during daily life's obligations, especially when we are busy or over-extended. Air is floaty and moves in chaotic patterns. When you feel distracted, dissociated, or preoccupied, you have too much of the air element. The stillness and stability of the earth and the heaviness of water can help balance too much air. You can achieve equilibrium by getting extra sleep, doing the Root Chakra Ritual (see page 176) or going on a nature walk.

Many of the concepts and recipes in this book are rooted in Ayurveda, which means science of life. It is an integrative medicine and life philosophy based on sacred Vedic texts. In

Ayurveda you have a unique dosha, or elemental profile, a body-mind-spirit blueprint to help you tailor your diet and lifestyle. Your dosha is a composite of elemental qualities of water, air, earth, fire, and ether. Look online for a dosha test and find out what elements are a part of your natural blueprint. I recommend *www.banyanbotanicals.com/doshaquiz*. Use this information to balance your chakras.

For example, the fire element wakes you up in the morning, helps you digest a meal, fuels your purpose, and helps you focus. When your personal fire is out of balance, you may be angry or frustrated or have inflammation or hot flashes. To achieve a better balance, you can increase attention to the cooling chakras: earth in the root center and water in the sacral center. Understanding the ancient system of Ayurveda and chakras can support you to live a life that honors exactly who you are and where you fit in your community, all of humankind, and the planet.

Why Chakra Tonics? Many of the spiritual, mental, and physical ailments that plague us can be reversed or stabilized with a healthy lifestyle. Men and women who eat a balanced diet, do not smoke, consume moderate amounts of alcohol, maintain a healthy weight, and exercise regularly live ten years longer than those who don't. Yet 70 percent of Americans report that they are not following a healthy lifestyle and say they don't have time to exercise or eat well. Only one in eight Americans are metabolically healthy, according to one study.

Likely most people ignore many of the recommendations for healthy living not because they lack knowledge of what is healthy, but because they don't how to change the limiting beliefs that keep them in unhealthy habits. According to one prepandemic study, fewer than 3 percent of Americans follow a healthy lifestyle. And while the evidence is mixed on how the pandemic, negatively or positively, affected lifestyle choices, the disconnect between what we know to be healthy behaviors and what we actually do is very real. Studying the chakras and using timeless wisdom can help. As you learn more about yourself through your study of the chakras, you can grow as a person, explore what is deep in your soul, and tap into the power of your true nature. Knowledge is power, but the true power is in how you activate that knowledge, and that is what the chakras help us to accomplish. What if you didn't have to sacrifice what you love to be healthy? What if following a healthy lifestyle rewarded you with more happiness, well-being, and enlightenment than any short-term, unhealthy impulse could provide? This is the message of the chakras. As a yoga teacher and health coach, I have seen how successful my students are in adopting a healthy lifestyle and transforming the quality of their lives for the better. They have learned how to change their minds, hearts, and spirits by using the holistic structure of the chakras.

Chakras can help you organize your self-care, mental well-being, and emotional health. If you were going on a long road trip, you would need enough gas, a good map, and a well-packed suitcase. The chakras help you see the path of evolution, your personal journey, while most people are living their lives without packing a suitcase, filling up their tank, or knowing where they are going.

Attention is another precious asset. Technological advances have taken a toll on our ability to concentrate. Smart phones, smartwatches, and smart appliances, along with many other devices, are supposed to make life easier. Yet, numerous studies link excess screen time, computers, TVs, and smartphones with anxiety and depression. These devices and technologies are often obstacles, rather than tools, for enlightenment. Our devices are growing increasingly complex, addictive, and invasive. We need balance. Focusing on personal development through study of the chakras helps us stay on track in a world of increasing distractions and information overload.

In the following chapters, you will find in-depth explanations of each of the seven main chakras and an array of healing tonics and elixirs to accompany them. The updated version includes six new Chakra Tonic recipes. All of the elixirs in the book help balance the stressors of modern living by increasing the much-needed healing elements of earth and water. And they are natural, plant-based, and easily absorbable. Chakra Tonics strengthen general well-being and help you compensate for excess consumption of processed foods, overwork, lack of self-esteem, depression, and anxiety. Study this book, visualize your chakras, do the rituals, and make the drinks. The rewards will be rich; you will gain greater vitality and clarity, and you will align you with the most powerful fuel of all, your divine nature.

CHAPTER 1

the chakras

C HAKRAS, the plural of the Sanskrit word *chakrum,* meaning "wheel," are filters through which our soul receives
and broadcasts pure energy. Chakras are psychic centers that
do not exist in physical reality, but in a spiritual dimension
that defies logic and quantification. Nevertheless, chakras
have been studied and celebrated by many cultures for thousands of years. Through the chakras we filter life's daily events,
dreams, hopes, desires, fears, regrets, thoughts, and communications. They are the ultimate devices for storing, sorting, and
retrieving mind, body, and spiritual data. Yet understanding
how exactly the chakras work is not intrinsic to their function.
Like the plumbing or electrical systems in our homes, they
operate invisibly, behind the walls of our physical bodies.

Existing on a level beyond ordinary perception, chakras
serve to organize the psychological and spiritual lessons of
the human condition in a philosophical system. Each chakra
corresponds to thematic emotional and spiritual issues and
challenges that can be overcome in order to move on to higher

levels of self-mastery and fulfillment. Each chakra represents a spectrum of energetic frequencies that correspond to psychological and sociological stages of development that we continually move through on the journey of life. As we tune into internal reservoirs of power, we are internally empowered to deal with the specific life challenges of that energy center, or chakra, and as a consequence to live more whole, meaningful, and fulfilling lives.

psycho-spiritual function of the seven bodily chakras

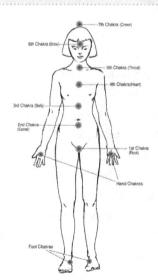

1st: Root Chakra: survival, basic sustenance.

2nd: Sacral Chakra: emotions, sexuality, procreation.

3rd: Belly Chakra: physical and spiritual power, body/spirit energy center.

4th: Heart Chakra: balancing center for love and affinity for self and others.

5th: Throat Chakra: center of eloquence and communication.

6th: Brow Chakra: clear mind and intuition center.

7th: Crown Chakra: transcendence, instantaneous knowing, divine connection.

Often lessons and situations repeat themselves through-out life. We begin our journey at the base of a steep and pointed mountain and then circle around and around to climb to the top. Along the way we continue to circle back to areas where we have been before.

What sets the chakras apart is that although they can be viewed as a psychological or philosophical organizational sys-tem, they are intimately linked to anchor points in the physi-cal human body. Unlike modern psychology and spirituality, the ancient Indian system of the chakras interweaves what Western science separates into separate disciplines. Psychol-ogy, physiology, sociology, even politics and economics are all linked by universal life force, which pulsates through the chakras of all living beings and drives the culture around them.

There are seven major chakras, each approximately two to three inches in diameter, lined up on the spine from the tip of the tailbone to the crown of the head. The locations of the chakras correspond with what science now understands as specific places along the spine where there are nerve plex-uses. Linking, the spiritual world and the material world, the chakras spin like pinwheels as they process and transmit energy from the physical realm to the nonphysical realm.

Responding immediately to the conditions of the mind, the physical body, and the unseen spiritual world, the chakras originally were understood experientially, in terms of ener-gy that moved through these psychic centers. The ancient

Hindu science of yoga viewed the *tattvas* or elements (fire, water, earth, air, and ether) as driving the life force in nature and the universe. The chakras were recognized as the body's most direct and immediate link to these elements. As the late Indian author and tantric scholar Harish Johari wrote in *Chakras: Energy Centers of Transformation*, "These elements are constantly coming and going with the circadian rhythms of the body. The ancient Indian science of Yoga therefore laid great emphasis on knowing these elements and on working accordingly, for the chakras are understood as playgrounds of the elements." The chakras are constantly in flux with one another, influencing in tandem our mind-body-spirit connection.

The immediacy of the chakras' regulation of energy has been connected theoretically for many years to the function of the endocrine system. The endocrine system consists of our ductless glands, which release hormones straight into the bloodstream; it is one of the body's great communication networks. These hormones act as messengers, and they are crucial and intrinsic to almost every function of the human body.

First discovered in 1902 by British scientists, who named them after the Greek word *hormo*, which means to set in motion, hormones directly affect nearly every function of the body. Many of the ductless glands correspond in location and function to the chakras and their energetic domain. For example, the butterfly-shaped thyroid gland, located at the front of the throat, corresponds energetically to the throat chakra.

In general, the chakras' locations and connections to physical health are as follows.

- ✦ Root chakra: Located at the base of the spine, it is associated with survival and sometimes the adrenal glands, blood, and overall general health.

- ✦ Sacral chakra: Located at the top of the sacrum. It is connected to the reproductive glands and the urogenital organs and the lower back.

- ✦ Belly chakra: Found at the solar plexus, it is associated with the adrenals, stomach, pancreas, and liver.

- ✦ Heart chakra: At the center of the chest, it is linked to the thymus gland, the heart, the lower lungs, the midback, and the shoulders.

- ✦ Throat chakra: Located at the base of the throat. Its function is enjoined to the thyroid, parathyroid, upper lungs, ears, and neck.

- ✦ Brow chakra: Between the eyebrows, it is also known as the third-eye chakra. Its physical correlation is with the pineal gland, the brain, the nose, and the eyes.

- ✦ Crown chakra: At the top of the head. It is associated with the pituitary gland.

Keep in mind that the actions of the chakras can be separated only intellectually. In the nonphysical plane, the function of each chakra often blends with the functions of others, especially with its neighboring chakras. Although there is much agreement on the knowledge of the chakras, there are some inconsistencies among students and scholars. In some cases, knowledge of the chakras has been passed on from student to teacher in a guru relationship. Western and Vedic scholars have created their own schools of thought. So have modern-day clairvoyants in many countries. Each has a personal perspective and many interesting things to say about the chakras. Since the existence and practical function of the chakras cannot at this point be scientifically proven, I encourage you to discern your own valid opinions regarding their processes.

The chakras direct streams of energy through channels called *nadis*, which run through the body conducting universal life-force energy. There up to 350,000 nadis, of which fourteen are considered primary. The three most important are the *sushuma*, *ida*, and *pingala*. The sushuma runs along the line of the spine and is the body's main energetic power line. In addition, the ida, or feminine stream, associated with the moon, and the pingala, the masculine *nadi*, associated with the sun, weave in and out of the chakras, creating polar streams of energy that spin the chakras in a clockwise rotation.

The image of these channels is mirrored in the caduceus, the internationally recognized symbol of medicine.

The chakras contain infinite color and energy frequencies, as they serve to process endless streams of data. At times the physiological or psychological flow of energy gets clogged and slows or comes to a standstill. When the chakras are slow, we may feel lethargic or shut down. When they are overdilated, processing or rotating at excessive speeds, we may feel vulnerable or spunout. We are "in the zone" when our chakras spin perfectly, like whirling multicolor pinwheels whose hues appear separate when still but become one in motion.

I use the analogy of a pinwheel because, likewise, the chakras have many colors that blend as they spin, and for each chakra there is a symbolic color that appears most often when the chakra is healthy, open, and vibrant. The chakras organize our inner light into the frequencies of a rainbow: the root chakra appears, red; the sacral chakra, orange; belly chakra, yellow; heart chakra, green; throat chakra, blue; brow chakra, purple; and crown chakra, violet or white.

cords: communication lines between people and their chakras

As processing units, chakras work like phone lines or e-mail. We can connect to others through our chakras, creating energetic lines, or cords, between our own chakras and those of other individuals. Individuals may also connect to whole groups, such as a teacher connecting to all of his or her students.

The communication cords that connect you to other people will hook up to chakras that correspond to the nature of communication occurring. For example, lovers may communicate from heart center to heart center, or they may set up lines connecting both parties' sacral chakras. Business partners may attach at the root chakra when discussing economics or join together through brow chakra connections when speaking about their visions for the company. Just as with our phone lines or e-mail, we may jam up or receive a virus.

In intimate relationships, we may leave connecting cords open at all time. These cords feel familiar and comforting—until one party disconnects them. When multiple chakra cords are suddenly broken in an intimate relationship, the human experience is heartbreak.

Chakra cords can facilitate communication, but they can also be misused. A person trying to manipulate another may drain a person's personal energy through the chakras.

As we said, understanding the subtle mechanical workings of our chakras does not affect their operation. They will continue to function without our knowledge of them. Chakras operate on a hidden level, and often people wait until they have a physical, spiritual, or emotional breakdown before they explore alternative methods of healing like balancing the chakras. Nevertheless, understanding the chakras can be a tool to assist in healthy physical and spiritual living. As we grasp our spiritual, physical, and psychological challenges and how they are interrelated through the model of the chakras we can become empowered.

In our efforts to understand the chakras, we often explain them in terms of three-dimensional models. While models lend tools for mapping the chakras and their activities, we cannot possibly be conscious of the level of information being processed through them. The chakras process and digest every thought, emotion, experience, and sensation each of us experiences. In this way they are somewhat analogous to extremely powerful computers with Internet service. The chakras store and process information and are connected to other chakras through a network of universal life-force energy. Yet this, too, is perhaps a poor model of their unfathomable complexity.

bija mantras

Repeating the sacred syllable and pondering its meaning
lead to its understanding. It is then that one understands
the self and gradually clears inner obstacles.

—Yoga Sutras of Patanjali, 1:28–29

The Sanskrit bija mantras are single-syllable mantras that introduce the primary sounds of each chakra, such as *Om*, *ham*, *lam*, and so on. The bija mantras work on deep levels to tune the chakras and have always been an important component in the energetic maintenance of the chakras in ancient Indian philosophy. "Sanskrit [is] a language of Cosmic consciousness," writes Jay Deva Kumar in *The Sacred Language of Yoga*. The fifty letters of the Sanskrit language are encoded into the petals of the first six bodily chakras from the muladhara (root) to the ajna (crown). Medieval schools of tantra believed that the letters of the Sanskrit language held certain powers and that by chanting them these could be accessed.

The bija mantras complement the Chakra Tonics and are the seeds from which more complex yet related mantras spring. Simple and essential, bija mantras are the easiest to pronounce and recite. "The plant transmits the seed-energy of nature into the body; the mantra transmits the seed energy of the spirit into the mind," write Dr. David Frawley and Dr. Vasant Lad in The Yoga of Herbs. The bija mantras are a great launching point for the study of mantras. For a more in-depth study of mantras correlating to the chakras, listen to Harish Johari's Sounds of the *Chakras* or *Chanting the Chakras* by Layne Redmond.

• •

In our modern age, as technology evolves to a new level, we are in turn accelerating the pace of our energetic bodies. Information is spreading at accelerating rates through the Internet, mass media, and other means of communication. There is more travel around the planet, too, resulting in deeper communication and better understanding among peoples. Chakras must "keep up" with the bombardment of all these copious amounts of data. The irony is that in this quickened pace we are too rushed to eat healthy food when we need it most. We are so busy that we forget drinking high-quality liquids and eating nutritious foods are exactly what we need to help us process the high levels of information and life-force energy that are being channeled through our bodies. With care and compassion, we can commit to a ritual of creating vital, fresh, and healthy foods, as well as drinks. In this we can offer our bodies as vessels for transformation and higher consciousness.

equipment

Y OU WILL NEED the following equipment to make the teas, tonics, and smoothies in this book.

blender

A blender can be used to puree solid ingredients such as ice, fruit, vegetables, or nuts. It can be used to make nut milks or simply to blend ingredients in smoothies. A powerful, reliable blender works best; however, techniques and ingredients can be modified to suit the blender. If you have a less powerful blender, ice can be crushed in a towel with a mallet or a rolling pin. Fruit can be cut into smaller, more manageable pieces. Also, your smoothie can be enjoyed on the chunky side. While a professional blender like the Vitamix works wonders, smaller, more portable ones can be handy and suitable for the job. I have a battery-operated camping blender, purchased at a garage sale, that I use on occasion that prepares simple soft-ingredient smoothies beautifully.

juice extractor

An investment in a juice extractor will significantly change the quality of your life for the better. There are several types of juicers available with various features and prices. A juicer should be easy to operate, dismantle, and clean.

There are several different extraction methods used in juicing. Centrifugal extractors cost less, and they get the job done. This type of juicer finely grates food and uses centrifugal force to expel and extract the juice into a container. The motors on centrifugal extractors have a tendency to add oxygen to the juice, which destroys vitamins, so juice from these extractors should be enjoyed immediately.

Masticating extractors are slightly higher-end machines. This kind finely grates and then "chews" the fruit or vegetable, creating even finer particles, from which it then extracts the juices. These high-quality juices will last up to one day in the refrigerator.

Hydraulic press extractors are the most efficient and expensive of juicers. The Champion Juicer is a hydraulic press extractor and is the choice of most professionals. This model uses revolving cutters to grate then crush any fruit or vegetable; then it places the pulp under tremendous pressure, creating juice that contains the highest nutrient content with no oxygen. This juice can be stored one to two days in the refrigerator.

A juicer will quickly pay for itself if you are purchasing fresh juices several times a week. For families with children, it is a wonderful way to ensure picky eaters receive their daily servings of fruits and veggies. If you want a juice today, but don't yet have a juicer, many juice bars will custom-make blends for you. Take a recipe from this book and they will usually juice à la carte.

Citrus juicers are used to extract juice from section fruits such as lemons, grapefruits, and limes. The least-expensive models depend on your muscle power to press the juice out. Citrus juice presses use pressure applied through a lever to remove the juice, and motorized juicers turn a ridged dome so that the juice will be extracted and strained.

grinder

Electric coffee grinders are a handy tool, great for grinding nuts or seeds into a fine meal or powder, rendering them easy to blend into drinks and often more digestible. Native Americans ground acorns on large stones. You will need a designated seed and nut grinder, as coffee residue is oily and the flavor will not easily clean out of a grinder.

oxo mini angled measuring cups

Brand names are usually not worth mentioning in kitchen measurement tools, but this cup is a gem for measuring exact quantities of small amounts of liquid ingredients between one and four tablespoons. If you use a spoon, you are more than likely to spill or overpour. The Mini Angled Measuring Cups come in sets of three and feature a patented angled surface that lets you read measurement markings by looking straight down into the cup. Oxo also makes a wonderful, reasonably priced flaxseed grinder and nut choppers.

tea-making equipment

+ French Press: Lovely for tisanes made with fresh-picked herbs because you can see the herbs floating in water.

+ Tea Ball or Spoon Infuser: A double-sided spoon or small metal ball that closes with a latch to hold dried herbs for teas, a handy, easy-to-clean way to brew tea with dried herbs.

+ Teapot and Strainer: Fresh or dried herbs can be immersed in hot or boiling water and then be strained prior to drinking.

◆ Individual Tea Bags: You can purchase empty small and large unbleached paper tea bags to fill with dried herbs to brew for chakra tonic teas. The t-sac filter is widely available online.

chakra tonics to go

Klean Kanteen manufactures inert steel bottles that hold twenty-eight ounces of liquid and weigh about five ounces. Designed by Robert Seals, a metal artist who felt surged with inspiration to eradicate the ubiquitous plastic water bottle after he heard a speech by Julia Butterfly Hill. After listening to Hill, the visionary eco-activist, bemoan the hazards of plastics on our bodies, souls, and environment, Seals set to work designing the Klean Kanteen. The Kanteen has a shape similar to an old-fashioned glass milk bottle, which deters bacterial growth in sharp corners. You can purchase Klean Kanteens to store your homemade hot and cold drinks at *www.Kleankanteen.com.*

CHAPTER 3

ingredients

"For this healing to be powerful, you must do it with great respect. Unless you have a spiritual relationship with the plants you use, it doesn't work."

"What was that lime drink you gave me earlier?" I asked next.

"Nothing but a good dose of spirit and lime," he answered with a chuckle. "You wanted to learn about the garden and my healing work, didn't you? Then you must experience the Earth and it's plants with your heart, not just your mind. That's the difference in our medicines. My medicine has magic in it, yours does not. Spirit does the healing, not science. Science is good, it is knowledge. But spirit has the real power."

—CONNIE GRAUDS, *Jungle Medicine*

mYSTICS, SHAMANS, and astrologers all pointed to monumental changes that would occur at the dawn of the twenty-first century. In order to raise personal vibrations to accommodate the increased frequency of the planet, excessive use of processed and denatured foods must be eliminated. The irony is that we are moving faster than ever; we've never been busier. We're turning to processed foods for convenience, yet these denatured foods have a slower, lower vibration than vital, fresh foods.

In the 1950s instant and convenience foods were believed to be the height of modern living. However, the Ayurvedic tradition was never fooled. In the ancient Indian tradition such processed foods lack intelligence, and over time their consumption contributes to a decrease in brainpower. On the other hand, fresh ingredients have natural *chelta*, or inherent intelligence, and confer the same to those who consume them. Our supermarket shelves are filled with items that are convenient, instant, and sometimes—according their labels— filled with important vitamins and minerals. But according to Ayurvedic standards, they are stupid.

"We are what we eat," as the saying goes. When we are too "busy" to make fresh drinks, we end up gulping unhealthy, devitalized beverages. Consider making an investment in your life, your health, and your energetic well-being. Take time. Use the freshest organic ingredients possible. They will promote clarity, natural intelligence, and peace in mind, body, and spirit to assist in your own personal transformation, mirroring that which is occurring on a global level.

Let's look at the ingredients used in chakra tonics, as well as some extra ingredients you may use to supercharge smoothies and juices.

water

Water needs to be filtered of toxins. Solid carbon block filters are especially recommended; they will remove particle sizes down to one micron and take out chemicals and bacteria like E. coli. You can get one to attach to your tap under the sink. A granular active carbon block filter that attaches to a pitcher will remove some impurities, but will not be as effective as a solid block carbon filter.

Reverse-osmosis filtration is best suited for chemically toxic or hard water that is high in alkaline minerals like magnesium and potassium. In other cases, reverse osmosis leaves water far below a neutral seven pH. Likewise, distillation removes contaminants but also strips the water of naturally occurring alkalizing minerals, so these methods are not recommended.

If you have acidic water, it can be alkalized by adding a little fresh lemon juice. See side bar on alkaline water, page 125.

dairy ingredients

Yogurt gives body and adds protein to smoothies. Organic yogurt with live cultures is recommended. Soy yogurt can be substituted for those who are lactose intolerant.

Milk is believed to be an important builder in Ayurveda. You can use either cow's or goat's milk. However, most milk purchased in stores has been pasteurized and homogenized, rendering it difficult to digest. In the Ayurvedic tradition the best milk is raw and nonhomogenized. Unpasteurized milk can be boiled slowly to kill harmful bacteria. Carminative spices like ginger, cardamom, and cinnamon will make cow or goat milk and even yogurt easier to digest. If you are lactose intolerant, rice milk or soy milk can be purchased in health food stores. Almond milk is available in most health food stores also, or see the recipe on page 69.

protein powder

Whey protein powder is made from the protein in cow's milk, but it contains no cholesterol, no fat, and no lactose. There are several different brands to choose from. Be sure that the whey protein you use is not made from cows treated with growth hormones and does not contain chemical sweeteners. There are many excellent vegan protein powders including pea, brown rice, pumpkin, and hemp seed protein powders.

canned coconut milk

Coconut is considered a divine plant in the Vedic tradition. Canned coconut milk is made from the diluted cream pressed from the thick white flesh of mature coconut meat, it is available in most supermarkets, Asian grocery stores, and health food stores.

Young Coconut

Baal is the Indian name for tender young coconut. Its juice or water is naturally isotonic, with incredible healing properties, and it is widely consumed for good health in tropical countries. It is available in cans or boxes at health food stores, Asian grocers, or online. Fresh coconut juice can be obtained by purchasing a fresh, whole young coconut at specialty grocers or health food stores. Chop off the pointy pencil top with a meat cleaver or machete to make a hole in the tough outer coating. Be careful. It can be challenging to open the hard shell of a fresh young coconut. You can then pour out the juice or simply insert a straw and drink. The tender flesh inside the young coconut is heavenly and can be scooped out with a spoon and added to smoothies.

nuts and nut butters

Nuts, considered a superfood by Dr. Steven Pratt, author of *Superfoods Rx*, are high in calories. Packed with nutrition and healthy fats, nuts are a less acidic form of protein than animal products and dairy. In addition, researchers have found that people who eat a handful of nuts a day are 20 percent less likely to develop adult-onset diabetes. Because nuts have a large percentage of fat, they have a tendency to go rancid. Store them in the refrigerator to keep them fresh. Add nuts and nut butters to supercharge any chakra tonic smoothie. Tahini (made from sesame seeds) and cashew butter are high in iron. Walnuts are high in arginine, good for healthy blood vessels and to reduce high blood pressure

seeds

Sunflower seeds, pumpkin seeds, sesame seeds, and flax seeds (high in omega-3 fatty acids and lignins) are great to supercharge any smoothie or to sprinkle in your juice. Like nuts, seeds are nutrient-dense storehouses of calories and protein esteemed in many healing traditions.

tofu

Tofu is soybean curd. It can be bought in any supermarket and comes in various degrees of firmness. Silken tofu is a common smoothie ingredient; this form of tofu is soft and easily blended into a drink.

herbs and spices

Making your own tea with dried herbs will be less expensive and more expansive than purchasing packaged teas or bottled drinks. Many health food stores have a bulk herb section, where most of the herbs in this book can be purchased. In general, one teaspoon of dried herbs equals two teaspoons fresh herbs. Add an extra teaspoon if brewing in a pot. Organic Ayurvedic herbs, such as *tulsi*, turmeric, and *ashwagandha*, are available in bulk at *www.omorganics.com*. A farmer's market is also a great source for fresh, locally grown herbs for tea.

Growing your own medicinal and culinary herbs is an excellent way to get in touch with the universal life-force energy in plants. In the Vedic tradition, plants convert the energy of the sun, which is pure universal life force, into something animals and humans can consume. You can check out what plants are available at your local nursery or order potted herbs or seeds online. When you grow your own herbs, make sure to plant in excess of your usage so that you do not destroy the plant when you make your teas and tonics.

You can order fresh, organic, wild-crafted bulk herbs in season from Pacific Botanicals in Oregon. You must call ahead one season so that they can plan their harvest. Order a pound of seasonal fresh herbs and hold a chakra tea party. Pacific Botanicals also carries a wide selection of dried organic, wild-crafted herbs. *www.pacificbotanicals.com*.

Spices are also an ingredient that can be purchased fresh or dried. Use fresh spices when indicated—turmeric, coriander, nutmeg, cumin, cloves, tamarind, and lemongrass. Use fresh ginger and fennel whenever possible.

essential fatty acids

Essential fatty acids are important for hormonal balance, metabolism, brain and immune function, as well as many other body processes. A variety of fats, and a healthy balance of omega-3, and -6 fatty acids are required for optimum health. Ironically, most Americans are not getting enough healthy fats, especially omega-3 oils, and many nutritionists recommend supplementing. High-quality flax oil is the most potent known source of alpha-linoleic acid, an essential omega-3 fatty acid. Evening primrose and borage oils contain GLA or gamma linoleic acid, an omega-6 fatty acid the body may use in hormone production, fat metabolism, and insulin regulation. A variety of nuts and nut oils, as well as coconut oil have many health benefits. Processed fats, especially hydrogenated oils, should be strictly avoided. For more information about how to balance your fat intake, read *Eat Fat, Lose Weight* by Ann Louise Gittleman, or *Fats That Heal, Fats That Kill* by Udo Erasmus. Adding flax oil, evening primrose oil, borage, or other high quality oils will add many health balancing properties to your chakra tonics.

healthy sweets

Sweet foods increase the elements of earth and water and, therefore, have a grounding quality. Americans' fast-paced achievement-oriented lifestyles have led to general cravings for comfort, love, and stillness. Many of us are not even aware of our imbalances, yet turn to dessert to bring us the comforting qualities that Ayurveda tells us sweet flavors increase. How can we consume in moderation healthy sweets that satisfy the body and quiet the mind? One healthy way would be eating sweet juicy fruits, such as mangos, strawberries, dates, and pineapples, or sweet potatoes, sweet beets, and cherry tomatoes (actually a fruit). Besides eating whole fruits and vegetables, there are myriad alternatives to refined white sugar when it comes to sweetening drinks, cereals, and baked goods.

sweeteners

Avoid refined sugar, which lacks the rich trace minerals and B vitamins. These are present in many less-processed sweeteners.

Agave nectar is a natural fructose sweetener extracted from the agave cactus plant's pineapple-like center. The indigenous people of Mexico believed the ambrosial agave plant held sacred healing powers for body and soul. Agave nectar has two grades, light and amber. It pours easily and will not crystallize, making it the perfect natural sweetener for teas and coffees.

Jaggery is made from the sap of sugarcane or palm trees and is processed without the harsh chemicals used to refine sugar. Relatively obscure in the West, jaggery's healing properties are well known in Asia. It is rich in the alkalizing minerals magnesium and potassium and high in iron, and it is said to strengthen the nervous system and assist in detoxifying the upper respiratory system. Many Indians working in environments with highly toxic air contaminants consume jaggery and swear by its ability to ward off the affects of dust or smoke.

Most berries are naturally sweet, and strawberries, blueberries, raspberries, and cranberries are all packed with antioxidants, vitamins, and minerals. Use organic fresh berries whenever possible. Marionberry syrup is delicious in smoothies and high in vitamins and iron. It is a favorite sweetener of the Pacific Northwest region of the United States, made from a particularly sweet blackberry hybrid developed in Marion County, Oregon.

Another fruit useful as a sweetener is dates. Chopped dates make great natural beverage sweeteners. You may soak the dates for fifteen minutes to an hour before chopping in order to blend them into smoothies more easily.

Sorghum is a grass introduced to the United States from Africa in the early seventeenth century. Sorghum was not grown extensively until the 1850s, when it became a staple for rural American cooks at a time when sugar was somewhat rare and expensive. A favorite sweetener of the Seminoles, the extracted juice from sorghum is boiled down to create a flavorful sweetener containing iron, calcium, and potassium. In fact, many doctors prescribed sorghum as a supplement for these trace minerals before the advent of multivitamins. Organic Amish sorghum can be purchased at *www.mannaharvest.net*.

Maple syrup is made from the sap of the sugar maple tree, rich in potassium, calcium, and iron, this sweetener is revered for its healing powers in several alternative health classics, such as *The Master Cleanser* by Stanley Burroughs. The syrup comes in several grades, depending on how long the sap has been cooking. Grade A light amber is a gourmet's choice, due to its less pungent flavor. Grade B has a stronger maple flavor but is more nutritious. The darker the syrup, the more trace minerals present, making Grade B recommended as an ingredient in healing tonics.

Honey is another natural sweetener. The ancient Egyptians and Indians esteemed this delicious treat, believing honey had healing powers when taken internally as well as externally. Honey does have antibacterial properties due to its enzymatic content, but heat and light will reduce effectiveness. Ayurvedic texts warn that heating honey creates *ama*, or toxins, and recommends eating it raw or unheated. Do not feed honey to infants less than one year of age.

Stevia is a popular, noncaloric sweetener currently sold as a dietary supplement. This plant, native to Paraguay, was known by the appellation *kaa-he-he*, or sweet herb, by the Guarani Indians. Stevia is an excellent choice for those looking for a nonchemical, no-calorie alternative sweetener, especially diabetics and those who are following a low-carb diet.

Rose Water

Rose water can be purchased or made with fresh organic roses. You can use roses from your garden as long as you don't spray them with chemicals. To make your own, boil a half cup of purified water and pour it over one cup of fresh rose petals (red roses will make the water a pale pink color). Steep for fifteen to twenty minutes, then strain.

the three gunas

According to the Ayurvedic perspective, the universe is made of three gunas, or qualities, that exist in and influence all of life. These qualities, present in the foods and drinks we consume, also influence the way we prepare drinks and meals. The first guna, sattva, represents the creative process, the laws of nature, and the ability to use one's imagination and inspiration. A meal prepared with love, care, and attention has more of a sattvic quality. Rajas stands for action and can be fierce and aggressive. Someone rushing or multitasking would prepare a meal rajasically. Tamas symbolizes completion and often inertia. A tamasically prepared meal would be one that required little effort—a frozen TV dinner or an instant entrée. Sattvic foods are believed to be the foundation for higher consciousness. They are light, nutritious, and easy to digest. Sattvic foods create peace, clarity, and joy. They are recommended for those on a spiritual path. Rajasic foods are stimulating and unsettling; examples of rajasic drinks are a mochaccino or a Red Bull. A tamasic food would be french fries, and a tamasic drink would be beer. Chakra tonics in general are sattvic! You can enhance the sattvic quality of chakra tonics by preparing your beverages with love and attention.

CHAPTER 4

root chakra

a T THE BASE OF THE SPINE lies the root chakra. Known also as the *muladhara* chakra, meaning "foundation," it is our initial energetic connection to the planet and our physical body. The root chakra is associated with the earth element. In the embryonic waters, a baby's heart beats at a rate of 160 beats per minute. The moment an infant arrives to take his or her first breath, the heart rate plummets to seventy-two beats per minute. At this vibratory frequency, as Maya Tiwari explains in *Ayurveda: Secrets of Healing*, we begin to lose consciousness of all previous incarnations. The muladhara chakra is the base, or first, chakra and the most energetically dense. We must give up our memories of other incarnations to live in the slower vibratory frequency of the earth. As life begins, we first attach to our corporeal bodies through our muladhara chakra. As babies we learn what it means to survive, to eat, to breathe, to have shelter and health. How we are treated and taken care of when we are very young directly affects this chakra. When our immediate needs are met, we feel secure and in turn gain a sense of trust in the universe. These lessons continue throughout childhood. Adults with first chakra issues may consequently forget to take care of themselves, failing to remember to eat, sleep, or engage in proper hygiene. Throughout our lives we must tend to the needs of our body, for the physical supports the spiritual path.

the root chakra cord

Through the root chakra, mothers energetically connect to their children so that spiritual information regarding survival and safety can be transmitted. Although the physical umbilical cord is cut at birth, an energetic line from the mother's root chakra to the baby's root chakra continues until the child is at least in their teens. Mothers have been said to have eyes in the back of their head because they know when their children are in danger or acting up. It's actually because of the cord from root chakra to root chakra. An adopted parent will always consciously or unconsciously make this connection. If you are a parent, clear this energetic communication line with the following simple imagery. Notice a connection between your tail bone and your child's or children's. Allow a cleansing and healing liquid-gold energy to flow through your connection to your child. This energy cord is one of great importance; keeping it at a high vibration will make communication between parent and child run smoothly. Think of it as a phone line; the gold energy dissolves fear and worry, which is like static on this connection.

A clear communication can be especially helpful in understanding the needs of infants who have not yet developed verbal communication skills.

sadhana

Trauma or mistreatment by parents or caretakers can be healed or altered through what is known in Sanskrit as *sadhana*, which means an effort exercised toward achievement of purpose or practice. While the literal translation of sadhana sounds mechanical, it implies a practice of a healing nature. In the tantric tradition, sadhana refers to the path of liberation. Meditating, Reiki, gardening, playing basketball, singing, and yoga are all examples of sadhana that could lead to deep levels of healing with the correct intention—that is, when a person engages in these activities with the purpose of reconnecting to their inherent power. Sadhana will heal the trauma where we became disconnected from our essence in the root or other chakras.

If all goes well, children grow to be adults who feel physically secure and able to take healthy risks. Some with great *dharma*, or spiritual missions, in life, like Mother Teresa, Martin Luther King, Jr., and Mahatma Gandhi, felt so rooted in their connection to their life and their purpose that they gracefully put themselves in great danger without fear. Great courage may be accessed through being grounded and simultaneously connected to a higher purpose. Paradoxically, "The main problem of the child or adult acting from first chakra motivation is violent behavior based on insecurity. A fearful person may strike out blindly or senselessly," explains Harish Johari in *Chakras: Energy Centers of Transformation*. To be in touch with our root chakra is to value all life, including our own. As Gandhi believed, nonviolence may be the only way to rise above the attempts by insecure and violent people who try to control others from the root chakra.

The root chakra is also connected to the feet chakras, which are deeply connected to the vibratory frequencies of the earth. Dancing, walking, and running all engage and activate our feet chakras and in turn stimulate the root chakra.

The root chakra is also associated with material prosperity. A person with a strong root chakra will have a strong physical presence, regardless of his or her physical stature or strength. We may have great talents and ideas, yet if they are not strongly rooted to the earth, we will be distracted or fail to take action in order to manifest what we need in order to survive.

The muladhara chakra will open up when we are in impending danger and signal our adrenals to give us a burst of energy to escape. In ancient times our first chakra might have opened up wide and created an increased heart rate and heightened awareness when a hungry tiger was chasing us. In modern times the chakra opens wide when a car is speeding toward us. When a group of people feel threatened or insecure, it signals their adrenals and they experience panic and stress. Past events that trigger fear in the muladhara chakra are often used to control groups of people for political gain. This is why it is important for us to be collectively in touch with our root chakra. Ironically, the tremendous prosperity of the last 100 years has led to so much technological development that Americans have been disconnected from nature and the earth element.

kundalini

An important vital energy, Kundalini lies dormant at the base of the spine. Kundalin means "coiled," thus, Kundalini waits like a sleeping snake until awakened, when it appears like a twisting flame. Kundalini begins at the base of the *kanda*, meaning "bulb," which represents the lower three chakras. The Kundalini heats up the lower chakras, which burn like a cooking fire under a pot of stew, releasing healing energies into the upper chakras. It may be awakened through spiritual practice, and because Kundalini is a powerful energy that bridges the body-soul connection, many spiritual aspirants attempt to activate its power. Yet Kundalini often remains elusive, sometimes awakening during an illness with a fever or a *kriya*, a rapid spiritual awakening, sometimes following dramatic or unexpected events. This may be followed by sleepless nights that are a result of Kundalini energy burning through the body, attempting to heal and integrate dramatic change, shifts of consciousness, or information. Originating in the muladhara chakra, Kundalini uses the polarity of female and male creative energy to drive it up the central channel of the spine, or the sushuma nadi. Kundalini may be activated through spiritual practice, but it cannot be invoked through sheer will or force.

. . . .

Many spiritual leaders have indicated that this is a time of great change and point to the year 2012 as one of great significance and the culmination of these changes. The world is changing its recipe for manifestation from two-thirds physical exertion and ⅓ energetic effort to the reverse. As tremendous changes arise in the planet, modern sages tell us we will only need ⅓ physical application and ⅔ spiritual stimulation. Economy of effort is important in the lower chakras. Simple healthy routines of taking care of our bodies, such as eating breakfast, will help unite body and soul in the upcoming planetary changes.

Protein grounds us and connects us to the earth. Many of the protein drinks can and should be taken for breakfast. Beginning the day connected to Mother Earth and the earth element allows the energy to blend and travel upward through the chakras for inspiration.

••• prana rising (rhubarb smoothie) •••

Originally from China, the rhubarb plant has unusual characteristics. It is a member of the chard family, but its leaves are inedible
due to the high oxalate acid content. Its bright red color and long
stalk suggest its connection to the earth and the upper chakras.[1] In
the ancient Persian religion Zoroastrianism, the first human couple
sprang from a rhubarb stalk. Rhubarb has been a plant used in many
Asian healing traditions and is said to assist in raising the energy up
from the root through the spine and the sushuma nadi. Its unusual
flavor will help us transform our energy from a more material level
to one that is more spiritual. Pregnant women and infants should
not consume rhubarb due to the high level of oxalic acid.

- 1 stalk of rhubarb
- ½ cup orange juice
- 2 tablespoons maple syrup
- ½ cup plain organic yogurt
- ½ cup strawberries
- ½ cup purified water or more orange juice
- (optional) Pinch of cinnamon

Cut the rhubarb stalk into several 2-inch pieces, place in a pan with
the orange juice and maple syrup. Cook mixture of orange juice,
rhubarb, and maple syrup in a nonmetallic saucepan (rhubarb will

---

1 Gurudas, The Spiritual Properties of Herbs (San Rafael, CA: Cassandra Press,
   1988).

react with metal) 10–15 minutes or until rhubarb is soft. Allow rhubarb mixture to cool. Place in a blender with plain organic yogurt,
strawberries, water (or more orange juice) and a pinch of cinnamon.
Substitute almond milk for yogurt for the vegan version. Blend at
high speed and enjoy!

rhubarb base

For a rhubarb base that you can set aside:

- 6 stalks of rhubarb
- 3 cups orange juice
- ¾ cups maple syrup

Cook in a saucepan 15–20 minutes and then refrigerate. This sweet
sauce can be used for smoothies or poured over fruit, yogurt, or ice
cream for an unusual desert. In smoothies use ¼ cup per serving.

prana rising in the raw

If you don't eat cooked foods, juice 3 stalks of rhubarb and 2 apples.
(Juiced rhubarb is said to assist in releasing the heavy energetic
load of TV programs and video games, and balances intuitive and
analytic energy.)

••• throw yourself on the ground •••

This mega-nutritious liver, kidney, intestinal cleanser will root you
to the ground. Beet juice, high in vitamin and mineral content,
cleanses the blood and activates the *apana vayu,* or downward move-

ment of prana. Mother Earth's red color resonates at the frequency of the root chakra and our first mother. In this juice you consume more fruits and vegetables than some get in a week. The American Cancer Society now recommends a whopping nine servings of fruits and veggies a day. With Throw Yourself on the Ground you qualify in one fell swoop. Christie McClelland of Gayatri Healing contributed this recipe.

- 6 carrots
- 1 red beet
- ½ lemon
- ½ bunch parsley
- 1 stalk celery
- ½ cucumber
- ½ red pepper
- (optional) Ginger and garlic to taste

Juice and enjoy with wild abandon.

⁕⁕⁕ beet soup ⁕⁕⁕

As more and more people begin to raise their awareness of health and healthy habits, I predict that more raw-food chefs and health advocates will be known, like Shazzie, on a first name basis. Glamorizing detoxification and healthy living, the British author, Shazzie contributes this recipe, excerpted from her book, *Detox Your World*. Beet soup not only includes an encore of the root-chakra-food beets, but also tomatoes, a superfood. Both tomatoes and beets are incredibly alkalizing and rich in vitamins and antioxidants. Tomatoes contain the rare and potent antioxidant, lycopene, plus potassium and vitamin C, among other nutrients, which gives them star-billing superfood status. Served with energizing, phytonutrient-dense macadamia cream, this alkalizing soup is the perfect meal when you feel spaced out or stressed out. Its energetic and nutritive qualities ground you and oxygenate your system, creating a more positive and realistic outlook on life.

- 1 medium red beet
- 3 strawberries
- 1 tomato
- 2 cups filtered water
- 5 spring onions (scallions)

Chop all solid ingredients and process in a blender with the water until creamy. If you like, you can strain it and add some of the pulp back in to get the consistency you like. Swirl in a generous helping of macadamia cream (see following recipe).

macadamia cream

Macadamia nuts contain omega-3 fatty acids that help to thin the blood, one of the body properties of the root chakra. Shazzie, author of *Detox Your World*, also contributed this recipe.

- 10 macadamia nuts
- 1 orange, juiced
- 4 small dates or 2 large dates, pitted

Add all ingredients to a coffee mill and blend until totally smooth. This might take several goes, depending on the power of your mill. Add to soups, dressings, or smoothies when desired. It also is good served on top of fruit. Make enough for two days and stir if needed before use.

healthy sodas

The public is more health conscious than it was ten years ago. The beverage companies are using this health trend to sell drinks that claim to be good for you. These drinks are full of herbs like echinacea, ginseng, and astragalus, but when you read the ingredients, the first on the list is high-fructose corn syrup, which is absolutely not good for you. Making your own sodas is simple and so much healthier. Simply make a tea, add honey or sugar and seltzer water to taste. Our bodies are made of up to 80 percent fluid. What we drink matters. Childhood diabetes has skyrocketed and obesity rates have increased by 50 percent in the last ten years in the United States. Sugary drinks contribute to the epidemic rates of these diseases. Don't let your children drink sodas; teach them how to make teas with honey and seltzer water. Set up a soda bar in your home, where kids can have a variety of herbs and juices to choose from for making their own sodas. Written by Kami McBride.

. . . .

◦◦◦ root chakra soda ◦◦◦

Herbalist and metaphysician Kami McBride submitted this fabulous alternative to commercial soda—a soda that tastes good and is actually good for you. This homemade spritzer includes ginger root—which in the Ayurvedic tradition is called "the universal medicine" for its comprehensive healing properties—and sassafras, another root plant native to the United States known for its cleansing properties. Orange peel contains rare and powerful citrus flavonoids, including hesperidin.

- 2 cups water
- 3 slices fresh ginger root
- 1 teaspoon dried sassafras root
- 1 teaspoon dried orange peel
- ⅛ cup honey
- 1 cup seltzer (carbonated) water

Put herbs and water into a stainless-steel saucepan. Bring to a boil. Turn off the heat and let sit for 20 minutes. Strain the herbs out, add honey, and let cool. Once the tea has cooled you can add seltzer water and ice. You can triple the recipe and store the tea in the refrigerator for up to four days and add seltzer water when you are ready to drink it.

When you crave commercial sodas, enjoy the cleansing and grounding benefits of Root Chakra Soda.

⚬⚬⚬ heaven on earth almond milk ⚬⚬⚬

Almond milk has a long tradition as a healing drink consumed by spiritual seekers and vegetarians, including vegetarian monks and nuns living in the cloister in the Middle Ages. It is an incredibly light, nutritious, delicious, and easily digestible form of protein. Also an alkalizing form of protein with easily digestible calcium content, it's a wonderful drink for vegetarians and anyone needing more protein in their diet. Pregnant women, especially in the last trimester of pregnancy, when the need for calcium and protein remains high and digestion may be sluggish, can benefit from fresh Heaven and Earth Almond Milk. Use it to replace soymilk to avoid phyto-estrogens, or plant compounds that mimic estrogens, which some believe disrupt endocrine function among other dangers and are implicated in female hormonal imbalance. Although much fear has been placed on almonds as a fattening food, studies show that almonds lower cholesterol and do not cause weight gain.

- 1 cup raw organic almonds
- 4 ½ cups purified water

- (optional) 1 teaspoon vanilla
- (optional) 1–2 tablespoons agave nectar

Soak the almonds in 3 cups of the water for no less than 1 hour, but up to 8 hours. After soaking you can either add the nuts to the blender unblanched, or you can enjoy the practice of peeling them. Pinch the almond between your hands to remove the skin or peel it off with clean nails, the almond skins should come off easily. Think of peeling almonds as a sadhana, or spiritual practice, to help you create heaven on earth in your daily life. In Heaven and Earth Almond Milk, the skins leave a slight bitter taste that is lessened if you strain the pulp from the milk, but it's delicious either way. Take the soaked almonds and half of the water they have been soaking in and place it in a blender. Add 1½ cups purified water to the nut mixture. Blend at a high speed 1–2 minutes. You can leave the almond pulp in the milk for extra fiber, or you can strain it through a fine filter like a coffee filter. Enjoy alone or add a fruit or vegetable. Sweeten the Heaven on Earth Almond Milk with 1–2 tablespoons of agave nectar. For richer almond milk, use a ratio of 2 parts water to 1 part almonds or for lighter almond milk use 4 parts water to 1 part almonds.

Fresh almond milk will assist in grounding the earth element in the body, but will allow the energy to rise up through the chakras.

bija mantra

The bija mantra for the root chakra is Lam (pronounced LUM).

bach's rescue remedy

Any serious accident, big emotional upset, or injury may disturb the root chakra connection. When this happens, use Bach's Rescue Remedy as directed in The Bach Flower Remedies by Dr. Edward Bach. He discovered that the vibration of flowers was stored in the water that formed morning dew. The healing frequencies of flowers contained in the Rescue Remedy are said to address the residue of unsettling emotions following trauma. Add several drops to water or juice and sip slowly.

which tonics do you need most?

Ancient Indian philosophy states that "all disease is linked to a disconnection with god force," according to Ayurvedic consultant and Sanskrit scholar Jay Deva Kumar. Emotional or energetic imbalances are the first sign of our disconnection to this "god force" and are best treated by chakra tonics. Which chakra tonic do you need today? The following list of questions can help you decide. In the case of serious physical or medical conditions, always consult with a medical doctor or health care provider.

Muladhara Chakra. Are you feeling spaced out or disconnected? Have you recently experienced a trauma that leaves you feeling separated from your body? Do you feel out of touch with the material world? Are you experiencing financial difficulties? If you answered yes to any of these questions, a root chakra tonic could help realign your connection with the earth element and your primal connection to the material world.

Svadhisthana Chakra. Are you feeling overly emotional? Or, on the other end of the spectrum, emotionally blocked? Are you feeling alienated from your sexuality? Are you feeling overly sexual in an addictive way? Are you afraid of destruction or letting go? Use sacral chakra tonics to help balance the water element associated with emotions and sexuality.

Manipura Chakra. Are you feeling egoless or egotistical? Do you feel that you've been forcing your will on others? Are you procrastinating on an important project or life goal? Use belly chakra tonics to help you balance the fire element, which helps you take action in the world.

Anahata Chakra. Are you feeling judgmental toward yourself? Are you feeling anger or upset toward close family or friends? Do you feel like you need to look at the world with more compassion? Heart chakra tonics help you balance with the air element and tune into compassion and unconditional love for self and others.

Vishuddha Chakra. Are you having trouble speaking your truth? Are you avoiding expressing important issues at work or in an important relationship? Did you recently realize that you talk more than you listen? Are you feeling stifled in your self-expression? Use throat chakra tonics to help you integrate the ether element into your life and help assert and express your personal truth without fear or judgment.

Ajna Chakra. Do you need more inspiration in your life? Have you been thinking about making major changes in your life or career that would be more in alignment with your higher essence? Have you been studying a lot or using your brain? Would you like to enhance your higher creative powers, like thinking outside the box or creating masterful art work? Use brow chakra tonics to help you balance the power of light and inner sight in your life.

Sahasrara Chakra. Do you want to enhance your meditation practice or increase your ability to connect to meditative states of mind? Would you like to experience yourself as soul having a human experience? Would you like to be able to quiet your mind and release mental chatter and mind clutter? Are you having trouble focusing your highest intentions? Use crown chakra tonics to balance the power of pure intention and cosmic connection in your life.

CHAPTER 5

sacral chakra

---

tHE SACRAL, or *swadhisthana*, chakra, is the concentric center of emotional, sensual, and sexual consciousness. Infants explore their surroundings and pure sensation from the swadhisthana chakra, frequently touching and placing objects into their mouths. Once the basic needs of the root chakra—food and shelter—have been met, the sacral chakra, represented by the color orange, takes over and governs the place where the impulse to create begins. Adults who live from the sacral chakra may seek to validate their vitality through their emotions or sexuality.

Like water, the sacral chakras elemental association, our emotions, sensations, and sexuality flow from a source—our higher essence. Water has a yielding nature, and sometimes it must be contained to unleash its power. In the same way, emotional boundaries can assist us on our spiritual paths. At times, however, like water, emotions and sexuality may gather too much power when contained, and judgment, when placed as a control to the powerful floods of energy that shower from the second chakra, frequently backfires. Affirmation of the powers of emotions and sexuality that arise from swadhista, or seat of self, serves as a more competent device to steer the tides of the sacral center. Emotions need to be validated for what they are. It is important to harness the life-giving properties of water, just as it is important to understand and accept the life-giving properties of emotion and sexuality in the sacral chakra. They are powers and tools to assist us on our sacred paths.

The lessons of this chakra are that you can merge with a group or others, but you must be able to honor your boundaries and reconnect to self. Bondings with others through sex or emotion are wonderful and satisfying; however, integrity of energy is key to this bodily energy chakra. In the upper chakras we can experience the interconnectedness of all people, but at the second chakra level, as physical beings, we all have separate lessons and separate physical bodies. The ability to discern when to open and close the second chakra is a valuable and important lesson. We may want to open up emotionally or sexually in friendship and romance. Yet the same energetic openness will not serve us as we walk through a crowd at a major-league baseball game.

Because the second chakra encompasses the creative act, the lesson of destruction is part of this chakra and reflects the powers of the goddess Kali, who is both creator and destroyer. Blockages in the second chakra may make us feel disconnected from our creative urges or unable to destroy or let go of our children, creative projects, or artwork. Healthy creativity contains a balance of manifestation and destruction. An example of this would be the creation of a beautiful sandpainting that is immediately destroyed by its creator, symbolically teaching release of attachment to creations. Children take particular pleasure out of breaking down sand castles, block towers, and other creations. Sometimes energetically powerful creators experience pain in destroying. Early parental judgment or societal conditioning that condemned destruction may render this side of the cycle of creation painful. In any case, this fear of letting go will manifest in distrust in the universe in the second chakra. Often highly creative individuals with these patterns will become hoarders. The dense vibrations of clutter may serve to keep energy in predictable patterns that block powerful surges of life force.

Another aspect of the second chakra is that it informs how we feel about our particular gender and procreation. Author Sonbonfu Somé explains that there is no word for sex in her culture, the Dagara tribe of Burkina Faso. Seen as a sacred act in which partners interact with the spirit world of the ancestors, sex becomes always a chorus of harmony linking the physicality of the lower chakras and the transcendence of the upper chakras. In most cultures, sex can be a purely physical release, or it may occur in communion with the higher levels of consciousness of the upper chakras. The second chakra's physical association is with the glandular organs of reproduction, the urogenital organs, including the kidneys, and the lower back, especially the sacroiliac joint.

A person who lives from his or her second chakra may be someone who gossips or frames his or her identity through relationship. Our bonds with others always have some degree of energetic merging, yet we must continually stake out our separate energetic territory on the sacral chakra level. Otherwise we surround ourselves with people who may not be the ones who support our higher spiritual purpose. If you are a hoarder, asexual, promiscuous, or fearful in relationships, your second chakra may not be running at optimum levels.

● ● ● sunrise juice ● ● ●

According to Ayurvedic texts, it is not recommended to skip breakfast, which many are in the habit of doing. When you skip this important meal, it is believed that you disturb *sadhaka pitta*, making you irritated and full of unsettling emotions. Responsible for bad hair days, the sadhaka pitta is a subdivision of the fire element. It influences our *get up and go* in the world, our decisiveness, and our spirituality. Ayurveda recommends fruit and vegetable juices for breakfast to balance sadhaka pitta. Ayurvedic texts go as far as to say that fruit in the morning is like gold because it is the optimum time to receive the nourishing physical and spiritual properties of fruit.

Sensuous, delicious, nutritious, and orange, Sunrise Juice will get you out of bed in the morning with a smile. It's filled with life-giving energy, and its sweet flavor will stimulate feelings of joy and contentment. Christie McClelland, yoga instructor, chef, masseuse, and founder of Gayatri Healing, contributed this recipe.

- ½ mango
- 6 tangerines
- 5 strawberries

Juice together and wake up to life. Take this cleansing, sweet, juicy fruit elixir 30 minutes before other breakfast foods such as hot cereal.

••• women's second chakra cordial •••

This delicious, sweet, soft elixir contains potent *damiana*, whose name comes from the Greek *aphrodisiakos*. Damiana acts directly on both the male and the female reproductive organs, making it an ideal sacral chakra herb. This cordial is designed for women, but can be shared with male friends, relatives, and partners. Roses, sweet dates, and apricots increase self-love, making it easier to share love with others. Drink this sensuous cocktail with a friend and enjoy the delicious power of the sacral chakra. Creation is sweet. This love potion also makes a great gift. Herbalist, healer and women's health advocate and author Kami McBride contributed this recipe.

- 4 cups port brandy
- 1 cup damiana leaf
- 1 cup rose petals
- ½ cup dried apricots

- ½ cup dates
- 1 teaspoon cinnamon
- 1 teaspoon cardamom

Put all ingredients in a half-gallon mason jar and let sit for 1 month in a cool, dark cabinet. Then strain all of the herbs and fruit from the brandy, using medium-thickness cotton muslin. Discard the herbs and fruit and put the liquid in a sterilized jar. This cordial will last for about one year. It makes a great after-dinner sipping drink, bringing warmth and nourishment to the second chakra area. Enjoy!

••• cayenne passion tonic •••

This simple supercharged tonic alkalizes the water element of the body, thereby acting as a cleanser for the urogenital organs. An ancient aphrodisiac, young coconut juice is enjoyed with cayenne and optional vanilla. This pH-balanced elixir will make you feel hot!

- 8 ounces young coconut juice, fresh or from a can with no other additives
- (optional) ¼ teaspoon vanilla
- pinch of cayenne pepper

Place juice in a clear glass, mix in vanilla, and sprinkle with cayenne.

••• fennel tea •••

This tea will release air or gas trapped in the gut. It's great for nursing mothers with colicky babies, as the tea will affect breast milk and have the same gas-releasing result for infants. Ginger and fennel are classic digestive tonics that assist the sacral chakra.

- 2 cups purified water
- 2–3 teaspoons fresh fennel (use the feathery green leaves) or one teaspoon dried fennel seeds
- 2 1-inch cubes of peeled ginger
- Bonus super ingredient: ½ teaspoon of dried burdock root—to increase the cleansing properties of this tea.

Boil water and pour over the fresh or dried fennel, peeled ginger, and burdock root. Steep for 10–15 minutes, strain, and enjoy.

••• sensual second chakra shake •••

Peaches have long been considered symbolic of sexuality and sensuality. The orange color of this shake reflects the cosmic aspect of the second chakra. This luxurious shake will inspire your senses and heal your body.

- 3 small or 2 large peaches cut into chunks
- 1 cup almond milk (see page 69) or plain yogurt or ½ cup plain yogurt plus ½ cup water
- Pinch of nutmeg

- ½ teaspoon chopped mint leaves
- ½ teaspoon ground cardamom
- 1 teaspoon finely chopped ginger
- 1–2 tablespoons agave or appropriate sweetener
- **Bonus super ingredients:** 2 tablespoons ground pumpkin seeds or pumpkin-seed butter
- 1 tablespoon flax oil for hormonal balance (flax oil is the richest source of plant-based omega-3 efas and high in lignins.

Blend and enjoy. Makes 2–3 cups. Pumpkins seeds are high in zinc, essential fatty acids, and plant sterols, and they are recommended for benign prostate enlargement, bladder disease, cystitis, kidney inflammation, and urinary pain, all related to the sacral chakra.

••• fall pumpkin smoothie •••

A sacred fruit and dietary staple for Native Americans, pumpkin is a superfood. High in fiber and rich in carotenoids, potassium, magnesium, and vitamins C and E, pumpkins are not just Halloween decorations, they are loaded with powerful medicine. Phytonutrients like beta-carotene and *alpha-carotene* have powerful antioxidant and anti-inflammatory powers, and the carminative spices in this smoothie make dairy easier to digest. The pumpkin's orange color and voluptuous shape make it an ideal second chakra ingredient.

- 1 can (8 ounces) pumpkin or 1 cup boiled or steamed organic pumpkin meat
- ½ teaspoons ginger
- ⅛ teaspoons nutmeg
- ¼ teaspoons cinnamon
- 1 banana
- ½ cup purified water
- **Bonus super ingredient:** 2 tablespoons pumpkin seeds

If using a fresh pumpkin, use a small one, as they are better for cooking. Cut the pumpkin open; remove seeds (you can wash and dry the seeds in the oven on a low temperature, 225 degrees.) Remove pumpkin stem, then cut the pumpkin into 2- to 3-inch squares of meat and skin. Steam for 15–20 minutes, until meat is soft. Scrape meat away from the skin. Use immediately or refrigerate for up to one week. Use one cup of pumpkin meat per smoothie. Blend all ingredients once pumpkin has been prepared.

••• sacred sacral juice •••

Honoring the sacred feminine power of the sacrum, the triangular shaped bone at the base of the spine, this juice unleashes the power of jicama, a root that's 90 percent healing, pH-balanced water content, high in the highly alkalizing mineral of potassium. The earthy signatures of root vegetables, like carrot and jicama, enhance the second chakra's water element and connection to the earth. Apples sweeten the brew and add the wonderful quercetin, a flavonoid with anti-inflammatory properties to the blend. This unusual yet delicious beverage will leave you feeling refreshed and in control of your emotions.

- ½ jicama, cut in chunks to juice or approximately 1 cup to ½ pound peeled jicama chunks
- 1 medium carrot, washed, not peeled, ready for juicing
- 2 small or 1 large gala or other sweet variety of apple, cut into chunks for juicing

Juice all items and then stir just before serving.

chakra tonic intentions

All Chakra tonics are liquid conductors of thought frequencies. When you focus your thoughts and intentions you can charge your tonics in a way that enhances their ability to effect the energetic frequencies of the chakras. In the book *The Hidden Messages in Water,* Masaru Emoto scientifically documents how the crystalline structure of water receives positive and negative thoughts and intentions, but we have known this for a long, long time. In the Ayurvedic tradition, it is understood that how you are feeling and acting will affect the preparation of food and drink. In fact, many ancient cultures understood the importance of blessing food with sacred intentions. Here are some of the intentions I use.

Root Chakra. I am deeply connected to the earth and nature. I feel rooted to the Earth, the universal spiritual mother. I am rooted to the earth like a tree (see also Tree Visualization, page 167).. Allow this chakra tonic to reconnect me with the Earth element. Drink your chakra tonic outdoors and contemplate the root element in all plants and trees.

Sacral Chakra. My emotions are an expression of my divine essence. I feel my sexual energy flowing freely in my body. I feel and validate my emotions and sexuality as a part of my divine expression on earth. I allow any imbalances to release so that I can fully express myself without excess in my emotions and sexuality.

Belly Chakra. I take appropriate action on my spiritual path. I drink in my personal power, the element of fire, which assists me in taking action in the world for my spiritual path. I take action as a part of my physical manifestation on earth. I allow my ego to lead me to right action. I release excess action and fire where my ego leads me to constant action without rest. I allow myself to rest and take action when appropriate.

Heart Chakra. I love myself and breathe deeply the element of air. My love of self allows me to love others. I use the element of air to love myself and others. My compassion for myself allows me to feel compassion for others. I experience divine and unconditional love on a daily basis.

Throat Chakra. I express myself as a soul having a human experience. I listen and speak my mind. I allow my spiritual truth to be expressed creatively and verbally without fear. I listen to others understanding that there are many truths in the universe, not only my own. I listen and assert my opinion when appropriate.

Brow Chakra. I clearly visualize my future as part of the divine plan. My visions are expressions of my soul. I use my intuition to help me make important and challenging decisions. I enjoy using the power of my creative visions.

Crown Chakra. I am a part of the divine plan. My actions are supported by the universe. I feel my connection to all beings and all of the cosmos. I am a part of infinite divinity. I am connected to a Supreme source.

bija mantra

The sacral chakra's bija mantra is Vam (pronounced VUM).

flavors and emotions

According to Ayurveda, tastes or flavors have elemental properties linking them to emotions. All foods and drinks have tastes, or *rasas*, which contain different qualities and have immediate effects on the mind-body. There are six flavors that can balance the body, mind, and spirit or throw it out of alignment: sweet, sour, salty, bitter, pungent, and astringent. Emotions have a parallel effect and correspond to flavors and their elements. For example, sweet-tasting beverages accentuate the earth and water element and correspond to the emotions of love and well-being. Sweet foods are often referred to as comfort food. Sour tastes, like sour emotions such as jealousy, are made up of the elements of earth and fire. "Sour grapes," or envy, may, on the positive side, alert you to talents or abilities that you are not allowing yourself to express or develop. Balance is essential to flavor and emotion, the right amounts can assist us in our spiritual and dietary journeys. Salty foods, like seaweed and potato chips, evoke the elements of fire and water. In a balanced amount, salty flavor can assist us in asserting our opinions; in excess, it renders us arrogant. Pungent flavors, like garlic, correspond to emotions like anger and aggression. Chili peppers, also pungent and comprised of earth and fire, are irritating to the belly. Someone suffering from acid reflux should avoid pungent emotions, for example. Grief is considered a bitter emotion, which in small doses can help one see the truth. The bitter flavor found in kale or collard greens enhances our ability to see truth and beauty in the ordinary.

Astringent flavors combine earth and air and can be found in cranberries, pomegranates, and crab apples. Astringency implies the satisfaction of simplicity and living within one's means. A popular bitter diet drink is unsweetened cranberry juice and flax seeds, which assists the dieter on a flavor/ emotional level by increasing the sense of fulfillment in moderation, thereby creating a decreasing emotional need for unhealthy foods, the foundation for long-term weight loss.

Most Americans eat a diet of mostly salty and sweet foods. Ayurvedic wisdom suggests balancing your chakras and emotions by consuming a variety of flavors.

belly chakra

THE BELLY CHAKRA, located along the spine at the solar plexus, is called the *manipura* chakra, meaning, "city of jewels." Associated with the element of fire, the belly chakra is our divine power plant or energy center. Fire fuels the will and tenacity needed to achieve our worldly goals. In Chinese medicine, the belly is signified by a written character that means between heaven and earth. This character signifies the duality of the manipura power center and the belly center's archetypical lesson of inciting the seeker to look beyond outer power toward inner power. The belly chakra kindles our desires to achieve, sparking the outer drive of the ego personality. Yet in order to attain true power we must also be able to simultaneously squelch the conflagration of the ego personality.

The art of surrendering to a higher power is not thought of as something of value in our culture. From an early age we are taught to be the best, to shut out the competition. As children, we learn to engage fully in the game of life, and it is natural for us to be emotionally involved and attached to winning objects and ideas. While this can lead some to great worldly success, it can also lead to misery. I remember speaking to a successful computer programmer and musician at a dinner party. He told me he did not like yoga because he couldn't win at yoga. This man had brains and artistic talent and could master many subjects in life; however, on a spiritual level he had not yet grasped the value of deeper personal power because he gave his energy to the outcome of his efforts. When people are always attached to the outcome of their work, then their "power" depends on that outcome.

Another truth about the manipura power hub is that there will always be plenty of people wanting to tell you what to do with your power and how. But each of us has our own power best suited for our own spiritual path. We must ignite our energy, engage our presence, and then let go of the outcome.

The comparing mind resides in the manipura chakra. Through it we compare ourselves to others and their accomplishments, attributes, and shortcomings. It tempts us to look outside for our power, to create a value judgment about whether we are "better" or "worse" than someone else. The irony is that when we turn inward we let go of our ego and its attachment to outcome, we can find our inner city of jewels, we follow our instincts. In the end, following our gut is infinitely more precious, valuable, and potent than any external source of validation.

In order to properly energize our bodies, we need a good diet, adequate rest, and exercise. The belly chakra governs the pancreas, adrenals, liver, and stomach.

••• chai masala energy drink •••

Build up your Manipura (belly) chakra with this blissfully delicious, blended drink. It combines potent anti-inflammatory ingredients with a traditional Ayurveda superfood: moringa. Chai Masala Energy Drink will help you boost your mood and generate prana when you have it in the morning. It wipes out inflammation that can lead to chronic pain and disease.

The ingredients here are bursting with goodness. This concoction contains natural electrolytes from the coconut water and monounsaturated fatty acids from the cashew butter (similar to those in olive oil) that can help regulate blood sugar. Packed with healthy fats like MCT, coconut butter has more of the immune-enhancing lauric acid than any other food besides human breast milk. Turmeric contains powerful nutraceutical properties, including the ability to decrease inflammation, fight cancer, and lessen symptoms of arthritis. Add 25 mg of CBD tincture to help further reduce inflammation or pain and modulate brain and nervous system imbalances.

- 1 cup coconut water, nonpasteurized preferred for flavor, nutrient, and electrolyte content
- ¼ cup cashew butter
- 3 tablespoons melted coconut butter
- 2 teaspoons chai masala powder (use a spice blend that does not have black tea powder)
- 1 teaspoon moringa powder
- ½ teaspoon turmeric
- **Bonus super ingredient:** 25 mg of CBD unflavored CBD tincture

Place the coconut butter in warm or hot water to melt.

Add coconut water to a blender, then add the cashew butter, melted coconut butter, chai masala powder, moringa, turmeric, and optional CBD tincture. Blend until smooth and creamy.

Raise your glass and enjoy!

··· fortifying fig shake ···

In the Ayurvedic tradition, figs and dates confer energy to those who consume them and it is recommended to eat one of each a day. Cinnamon is believed to lower cholesterol and is effective in treating diabetes, according to U.S. Department of Agriculture research.

- ¼ cup coconut milk
- ½ cup filtered water
- 2 large or 3 small figs cut in small pieces; use dried figs if fresh are unavailable
- 1 date, pitted and then finely chopped
- dash of cinnamon

Place all ingredients in a blender and puree at high speed until smooth and frothy.

··· be strong banana shake ···

This delicious and light elixir is based on a *jamu*, an Indonesian herbal-healing tradition recipe, combining the healthful spices tamarind and turmeric. Turmeric is a wonder herb. It has antibacterial, antimicrobial, anti-inflammatory properties. Tamarind and turmeric are naturally alkalizing spices. Validating the yellow hue of manipura, this high-potassium, energy-rich shake is great for a balancing breakfast or afternoon snack. Omit tamarind and serve to children.

- 1 banana cut in four pieces
- 1 tablespoon tamarind paste or pulp from a tamarind pod
- 1 teaspoon turmeric
- ¾–1 cup cow's milk, almond milk, rice milk, or soy milk
- 3 dates, soaked for 15 minutes, pitted, then sliced into little pieces for the blender (or substitute 1–2 tablespoons agave)
- **Bonus super ingredients:** Add 1 or 2 of the following:
  - 1 tablespoon sesame seeds—high in potassium, selenium, thiamine, and polyunsaturated fatty acids, great support for adrenals
  - 1–2 tablespoons maca powder, an adaptogen and natural hormone balancer, a great super ingredient for menopausal women
  - ½ teaspoon Ashwagandha powder, an Ayurvedic adaptogen and used in Indian medicine as ginseng is in Chinese medicine
  - 1 small vial Siberian ginseng or 1 tablespoon, use for adrenal support, do not use if pregnant.

Blend and serve!

jamu

Indonesians often begin their morning drinking a daily dose of jamu, which translated literally means "herbal remedies used internally and externally for health and beauty." The origins of jamu are difficult to pinpoint; however, many trace its genesis to the royal palaces, where Indonesian nobility received regular visitors from India, the Middle East, and China as a stop along the spice route. The foreigners brought their respective herbal traditions, which then mixed with local medicine. In theory this was the birth of jamu, which later spread to common people, and today around 80 percent of all Indonesians drink a daily jamu. Although some jamu is now mass-produced in pills or tablets, many people still consume jamu in liquid form. Often sold by local vendors who brew herbal remedies in their own kitchens and then sell them *jamu gendong*, which means jamu carried on one's back. Colorful bottles are sold door-to-door to health-seeking patrons who swear by the formulas, containing well-known herbs and fruits such as mango, ginger, pineapple, papaya, banana, garlic, and turmeric. Other concoctions contain more obscure herbs indigenous to the unique and diverse ecosystem of Indonesia. More than 40,000 species of plants exist in the rainforests of Indonesia. This country of many islands is the home of 10 percent of the world's total plant species and is considered one of the most ecologically biodiverse areas in the world. There is hope that in the vast assortment of plant life in Indonesia substances might be discovered to cure some of the degenerative diseases plaguing Western countries today, such as cancer, diabetes, or AIDS.

coca colonization

In the 1950s French communists coined a term to describe the pervasive and insidious techniques used by American multinational corporations to exploit less economically developed countries in marketing American products: Coca colonization. Although ostensibly this had nothing to do with health or spirituality, a subtle undertone to the marketing of American food and beverages implied that these countries' cultural ways of eating, drinking, and health care were inferior. Fifty years later type 2 diabetes and other degenerative diseases related to a poor diet, including a great deal of processed, chemicalized foods and carbonated sodas, have now reached epidemic proportions around the world, especially in countries where a Western diet has been adopted. From 1985 to the year 2000 a 500 percent increase in diabetes cases worldwide was recorded. Many overseas public health experts, including eminent Australian epidemiologist Paul Zimmet, point their finger at Coca colonization for this worldwide health debacle.

··· holy cow ···

Cow's milk, revered for its healing power in India, is consumed with
trepidation among the health conscious in the United States. According to Ayurvedic texts, cow's milk provides special and unique
nutrition unavailable in any other food, but it should usually not
be consumed cold. Instead, cow's milk is made more digestible if
boiled gently for five to ten minutes and blended with carminative
spices like cardamom and ginger. In addition, Ayurvedic tradition
recommends using raw, nonhomogenized milk whenever possible.
If you are a vegan, substitute almond or soy milk for the cow's milk.
Enjoy the healing medley of spices of this tonic, including turmeric,
an anti-inflammatory and anticarcinogen. Its bitter and sweet flavor
blends well with the milk.

- 2 cups unpasteurized whole milk or substitute regular
  milk, almond milk, or soy milk
- 7 whole pods crushed cardamom (or ¼
  teaspoon ground)
- 1 stick cinnamon (or ¼ teaspoon ground)
- 2 dates, soaked for 15 minutes to make them
  easier to blend
- ¼ teaspoon black pepper
- ¼ teaspoon turmeric
- ½ teaspoon finely chopped ginger
- 1–3 tablespoons agave or other sweetener (add more if
  not using soaked dates)

Bring cow's milk to a slow boil for 5–10 minutes with cardamom pods and cinnamon stick (if not using ground ingredients). If using almond or soy milk, do not boil. Heat almond or soy milk to a near boil, then add cardamom pods and cinnamon stick. Allow mixture to steep for 5–10 minutes. Cool slightly, strain and then put in a blender. Add the rest of the ingredients. Blend this hot mixture carefully for a minute or two on high. Pour and enjoy.

••• manipura manhattan •••

The alcoholic version sometimes contains digestive bitters, which help the third chakra assimilate energy. The fennel acts as a digestive tonic in this yogic cocktail named by yogi Nathan Lupo. Manipura Manhattan is especially good following a large meal or anytime digestion is sluggish.

- 1 small fennel bulb or 1 large bulb, cut in half
- 1 Asian pear (or apple if unavailable)
- 1 Bartlett or other sweet pear
- **Bonus super ingredient:** ½- to 1-inch chunk of unpeeled ginger

Remove the stem and a few of the outer layers on the fennel bulb, then cut in pieces suitable for juicing. Combine ingredients. Juice. Stir. Enjoy.

gem therapy

The ancient sages of Ayurveda studied and placed great importance on the healing properties of gems. Examining the different effects of stones on the body, they noticed how the colors and energetic qualities affected the human aura and the chakras. *Jyotish* is the Vedic astrological system that was once a part of Ayurveda and that relates gemstones to the planets in order to assist in balancing a person's astrological influences. Gemstones can be worn or actually consumed. Little known ancient Ayurvedic techniques for preparing gems for consumption are documented in the 2001 film *Ayurveda: The Art of Being*. Gemstones are burnt or crushed in exacting procedures that make them nonpoisonous and then taken as a powder in food or in drinks. Gem tinctures are a wonderful alternative to utilize the energetic powers of gemstones to open and balance the chakras. If your budget won't allow for a sapphire ring, gem tinctures capture the subtle essence of the beautiful stone in a water and alcohol solution that doesn't cost more than a movie. Gem elixirs are made by soaking gems in the water and alcohol solution for up to one month; then they are dispersed into tinctures. Caitlin Phillips has been working with flower essences and gem elixirs for the past ten years, using the subtle vibrations of minerals and plants to heal the chakras. She recommends adding five to ten drops of the following gem elixirs to your chakra tonic in order to increase it's potency.

The following are Alaskan Gem Elixirs available at specialty stores or at *www.alaskanessences.com*.

✦ Root Chakra: Malachite or ruby supports ability to ground and connect spirit to body.

✦ Sacral Chakra: Bloodstone stimulates release of built up emotions.

✦ Belly Chakra: Gold strengthens and balances for tapping into inner truths, joy, and wisdom.

✦ Heart Chakra: Chryoprase balances heart chakra to divine and harmonious unions.

✦ Throat Chakra: Azurite promotes communication with authenticity, vitality, and gentleness.

✦ Brow Chakra: Diamond aligns with divine purpose.

✦ Crown Chakra: Scepter Amethyst opens us to our highest potential.

Caitlin also recommends the chakra elixirs made by one of her favorite manufacturers.

Pegasus Products (*www.pegasusproducts.com*)makes custom blends of flower remedies and gem elixirs for all seven bodily chakras and an eighth chakra blend. Formulated to harmonize the frequencies of the corresponding chakras, a few drops of these liquid elixirs increase the effectiveness of chakra tonics.

••• licorice belly root tea •••

Along with flavonoids and isoflavonoids, licorice root has something called glycyrrhizin, which yields *glycyrrhetinic acid*, which is similar in structure to the hormones of the adrenal cortex. Licorice is also an excellent tonic for the digestive system. However, it will raise your blood pressure, and it acts like the hormone ACTH, causing you to retain sodium and potassium, so avoid this tea if you are pregnant or have high blood pressure. Licorice is also great for stomach ulcers (it coats the stomach wall with a protective gel, increases flow of bile, lowers blood cholesterol levels, lowers stomach acid, and relieves spasms of the large intestines). A great tea for those who suffer from acid reflux.

- 1½ teaspoon licorice root
- 1 teaspoon dried spearmint leaves
- ½ teaspoon slippery elm root
- 3 cups purified water

version 2 of licorice belly root tea—adrenal formula

This version is a great adrenal gland fortifier. It will give a light energy boost and soothe the belly. Good for recovery from illnesses.

- 1 teaspoon licorice root
- 1 teaspoon dried spearmint leaves
- 1 teaspoon astragalus root

- 3 cups purified water
- 1 or 2 teaspoons of agave, jaggery or other sweetener

Place herbs in a French press, teapot, or tea bag. Boil water and add to herbal blend. Strain if necessary; sweeten and enjoy.

••• papaya pineapple smoothie •••

Papaya is the "acknowledged universal healer" in the Indonesian healing tonic tradition of jamu. The enzyme papain seems to be able to digest almost anything. It is found in the juice of the fruit and is highly concentrated in the leaves of the plant. Pineapple contains the enzyme bromelain, which is also an appetite suppressant.

- ½ pineapple cut into small pieces
- 1 small papaya or ¼ to ½ large papaya cut into small pieces
- 1 cup apple juice or 1 cup purified water
- Bonus super ingredients: 1 teaspoon probiotic formula, or small vial of Siberian ginseng for adrenal support

Place ingredients in a blender and puree at high speed. Serve and enjoy this tropical cleansing/digestive smoothie.

... wild weed digestive tonic ...

Our physical well-being depends on healthy digestion and assimilation of what we consume and digest. This tonic tea helps keep
things moving in your lower chakras, supporting healthy peristalsis
and elimination. This tea focuses on the command center of your
nervous system, the belly chakra or Manipura. The recipe calls for
wild ingredients found in your backyard, a nearby park or natural
reserve, or wherever you can find fresh dandelion flowers and leaves.
(Do not forage in an area where pesticides have been sprayed.) This
tonic reminds us that we can find energy and lessons everywhere,
including weeds. Think about the paradigms or world beliefs you
may hold in your chakras. Don't let them hold you back. This tea
will help with your feelings, especially for those who feel too much.
It keeps the energy moving. Great for spirits who feel responsible
for the planet and all of the damage that humans have done to it.

Though it's possible to buy dandelion leaves at the grocery store
(flowers aren't generally sold in stores), this tea is best made after
foraging for wild dandelion.

- ½ teaspoon of anise seeds
- 2–3 pieces of one-inch crushed ginger
- Wild dandelion, yellow flowers and leaves, about 3–5
  flowers, 3–5 small leaves; if you only have one or the
  other, use 6 flowers or 10 small leaves

Crush ginger with a mallet or jar. Boil water, and place anise seeds and other ingredients in a teapot or tea press. Double the ingredients if you are making more than one cup! Steep, strain, and enjoy.

adrenal exercises

Excessive exercise overstimulates the adrenals. Avoid strenuous yoga flow classes. Instead, focus on gentle strengthening or stretching in yoga asanas. Restorative yoga is wonderful for adrenal burnout and stimulating the parasympathetic nervous system (slows heart and breath rate and reduces basal metabolic pressure). Other yoga asanas for the belly chakra are boat pose for strength and all forward bends for surrendering ego.

bija mantra

The bija mantra for the belly chakra is Ram (pronounced RUM).

heart chakra

OUR HEART CENTER, the *anahata chakra*, rules our soul's affinity with self and others, utilizing the elemental association of air. Love, like air, is all around us. The quality of the air we breathe and the breaths we take are associated with this love. When we take a deep breath, we truly love ourselves.

All of us have affinity for people, places, objects, homes, animals, and myriad other things. Often these affinities are inexplicable yet unique and important components of our beings and spiritual fingerprints. These affinities create desires that can guide us on our spiritual path or sometimes lead us to delusion. A balance in the fourth chakra, must be struck between loving oneself and loving others. Our love of others must flow from a strong and connected love of self.

The lesson of the fourth chakra is similar to the instructions for putting on an oxygen mask on an airplane. You must put on your mask first before you assist others. If we don't direct the same empathy, love, and forgiveness toward ourselves that we radiate toward others, we will suffocate.

Often people who have affinity with others but have trouble turning this affinity inward are afflicted with heart problems and sometimes heart attacks.

We are conditioned by education, family, and social pressures to succeed and to seek validation of our success from outside sources, so the dance between loving oneself and loving others is a complex one. For example, parents' wishes might be that their children have secure and reliable occupations. The children might honor their wishes and work as bankers or accountants or they may follow their hearts and study filmmaking or art.

This love of self reflects a person's sense of belonging and value in the world. People with closed fourth chakras sometimes feel like misfits because their lack of energy in the heart chakra blocks them from connecting with others. As we move to the anahata chakra, our struggle with internal power must dissolve in order to attain mastery of this chakra. The choices of the fourth chakra involve higher love and honor with our heart.

The fourth chakra is sometimes thought of as the first step toward transcendence or a stepping-stone out of the physical, sexual, and ego-oriented issues of the lower chakras. As we look at the chakras as power centers, the fourth can be seen as the center linking the more physical *kanda*, or bulbs, of the three lower chakras with the more ascendant lessons of the fifth, sixth, and seventh chakras. The heart can seem like an oasis, yet it is only a rest stop on the road to enlightenment—and at times a distraction.

When our heart center vibrates in affinity, we align with our spiritual path. Often animals and children are attracted to someone whose fourth chakra resonates healthy self-love. When in balance, we feel affinity for ourselves, and this reflects in our healthy self-esteem. This affinity deeply affects our immune system.

When we rely on validation to come from others, we may compromise or give away our power, and the same applies to our immune system.

We are called to do, be, and be with what is harmonious to our heart and soul. That is our dharma. If our life's work and life choices are not in harmony with our spirit, our work or our health may slip away from us. We must choose our physical roles in the world wisely, yet our work and roles in the world are simply the costumes that we wear for the costume party called life. Our souls know better, and when we take our costumes too seriously, we lose out on our lessons and a chance to evolve and go to the chakras above the fourth.

Physically, the heart center is associated with, of course, the heart, the overall immune function, the mid back, and the shoulders. Although physical immune function is rather complex, involving all of the lower chakras, the glandular association of the heart center, the thymus gland, plays a critical role in the body's immune response.

The thymus is a small gland, located under the breast-bone, that processes white blood cells into T lymphocytes. T lymphocytes work on many levels to defend the body against viruses, bacteria, and foreign and abnormal tissue. The thymus thrives on high doses of antioxidants and fruits and vegetables loaded with vitamin C, which assist it in defending the body against what is not in affinity with it as a system. Zinc and selenium are minerals that support the thymus.

... high-esteem kiwi quencher ...

The color of the anahata chakra is green, and kiwis, which have extremely high levels of vitamin C, are of this vibratory color. Vitamin C supports the thymus gland and the heart center as the primary center of immunity. This recipe has some bonus super ingredients you might try one or more of a powerful immunity boosters. *Chyvanaprash* is a *rasayana*, designed to restore vital energy. A super-concentrated blend of many herbs including *amla* berries, or Indian gooseberries, it is extremely rich in antioxidants. The jamlike paste, named after the Indian sage Chyawan, is an antistress and antiaging tonic suitable for almost anyone. The main ingredient, amla berries, have been used in Indian herbal medicine for thousands of years to strengthen immunity. Coenzyme Q10 is an enzyme great in combination with vitamin C; it is immune enhancing and has particular benefit in cardiovascular diseases.

- 4 fresh kiwis, peeled and cut in 3 pieces
- ½ cup raspberries, washed, preferably organic, use frozen if necessary
- ½ cup of orange juice or ½ cup water or ice
- (optional) 1 tablespoon Marionberry syrup or other suitable sweetener
- Bonus super ingredients: ½ to 1 teaspoon spirulina or any green powdered food
- 1 tablespoon chyavanprash, an ancient Indian sweet tonic paste
- 1 tablespoon liquid Coenzyme Q10 (check label for proper dosage as some brands may vary)
- Kumquats (optional for garnish)

Place kiwis, raspberries, water, ice, or orange juice; sweetener; and super ingredients in a blender. Blend 1–2 minutes on high speed. Garnish with sliced kumquats.

••• hibiscus rose water affinity tonic •••

This delicious blood-red tonic can be served as a hot heart warmer or a cooling ice tea. Hawthorn berries are excellent for cardiovascular health; hibiscus is high in vitamin C.

- 1 tablespoon ginger, 1-inch piece of ginger peeled and sliced thinly, or ginger tea bag
- 3 cups purified water
- 2 tablespoons hibiscus flowers
- 1½ teaspoons hawthorn berries
- ½ teaspoon rose water; purchase or make your own (see recipe, page 55)
- 1–3 teaspoons raw honey, agave, or other appropriate sweetener

If using fresh ginger, peel a 2-inch chunk of ginger and then cut into 4 pieces. Place into a pan with 3 cups purified water. Bring to a boil, then simmer for 10 minutes. Turn off heat and add hibiscus flowers and hawthorn berries. Brew for 5 minutes or more. Add rose water and sweetener. Serve warm or cool.

free radicals

Free Radicals are molecules that are missing an electron, resulting in a molecule that has lost an electron and becomes unbalanced and is reactive. Because the molecules have lost an electron, they try to "steal" an electron from other molecules, causing a chain reaction that moves quickly through the body as molecules "steal" electrons from each other in rapid progression. Antioxidants neutralize free radicals by donating one of their own electrons, ending the electron "stealing" reaction. Free radicals can be caused by environmental factors such as pollution, radiation, cigarette smoke, and herbicides. Free radicals can be made when oxygen and fat molecules react and some free radicals are created during normal metabolic processes. Normally, the body can handle free radicals, but if antioxidants are unavailable, or if the free radical production becomes excessive, especially when a person is ill or exposed to toxins, damage can occur. Of particular importance is that free radical damage accumulates with age. Putting out the fire of free radicals is one of the important steps you can take to slow down the aging process. Drinking antioxidant-rich fresh-fruit smoothies and vegetable juices can help the body deal with free-radical exposure from diet or the environment, and help slow the aging process by reducing acidosis and helping the body retain its slightly alkaline pH of 7.4.

⋅⋅⋅ **lemon balm tisane** ⋅⋅⋅

Lemon balm has a wonderful scent and has long been used as a spirit lifter, antiaging herb, and antidepressant. One of my favorite herbs to enjoy fresh. Buy a plant so you can use it all the time. Lemon balm is known as the herb of longevity. There are stories of people in Mrs. M. Grieve's *Modern Herbal* who lived to be more than a hundred years of age and drank lemon balm tea daily.

- 2 teaspoons fresh mint leaves
- 2 teaspoons fresh or 1 teaspoon dried lemon balm leaves—*Melissa officinalis*
- 3 cups purified water

Place ingredients into a French press, teapot, or tea bag, with boiling water. Steep for five to ten minutes. Strain if necessary and enjoy.

⋅⋅⋅ **carmelite water** ⋅⋅⋅

A variation of Lemon Balm Tea first made by Carmelite nuns in the fourteenth century, Carmelite Water uses the heart-warming qualities of lemon balm and angelica. It is a good tonic for heart and lungs and was believed to ward off evil spirits in more superstitious times. Lemon zest contains bioflavonoids, which strengthen capillaries, which in turn help deliver vitamin C to all parts of the body.

- 1 teaspoon lemon juice
- 1 teaspoon lemon zest

- ⅛ teaspoon nutmeg
- 1 tablespoon fresh lemon balm, or ½ teaspoon dried lemon balm
- ½ teaspoon dried angelica root

Once again, place ingredients into a French press, teapot, or tea bag, with boiling water. Steep for five to ten minutes. Strain and enjoy.

pranayama

One of the mechanisms that the body uses to control the blood pH is the release of carbon dioxide from the lungs. By adjusting the speed and depth of breathing, the brain and the lungs are able to regulate blood pH levels minute by minute. Ancient yogis understood this to be the yogic science of breath control, or *pranayama*. They believed that its practice would lead to elevated levels of prana, or life force, in the body. Scientifically, optimal breathing is alkalizing. Improper breathing can cause acidosis.

⋯ fresh air lemonade ⋯

Lemons contain sumptuous quantities of vitamin C to support the thymus and the immune system. You don't have to spend a fortune to stay healthy. You can make this simple but potent beverage with organic ingredients for a couple of dollars, but the payoff in overall health is great. Fresh Air Lemonade offers immunity support and is a great drink when you feel like your coming down with something. Also great for children!

Christie McClelland of Gayatri Healing contributed this recipe.

- 3 apples (I use fuji)
- ½ lemon
- 1 thumb-size chunk of ginger

Juice and drink immediately. Tastes just like lemonade without the added sugar.

••• hatha yoga tonic •••

- 8–10 ounces water
- ¼–⅛ teaspoon turmeric (turmeric is an excellent overall tonic for all chakras and for strengthening and increasing flexibility in the joints)
- 2 1-inch cubes of peeled ginger
- Optional zest of juice and ½ cup fresh orange agave, maple syrup or stevia to taste

Bring water to a gentle boil, place ginger in water for approximately 3–5 minutes. Remove ginger from the pan. Add remaining ingredients and stir.

••• power yoga tonic •••

- 8–10 ounces almond, soy, cow, or goat milk
- ⅛–¼ teaspoon turmeric
- ¼ teaspoon powdered ginger
- 1–2 teaspoons raw honey or agave

Gently heat the milk in a saucepan, add turmeric, ginger, and sweetener. Pour and enjoy. This is a good drink to consume half an hour before a vigorous yoga practice. The milk will help build muscle and tissue in the long-term and sustain you physically in the short-term.

hatha yoga

The ancient practice of hatha yoga has always been a tool for spiritual development and awakening or cleansing the chakras. *Hatha* in Sanskrit means "sun-moon" and Hatha Yoga refers to the physical poses of yoga. Although the yoga practiced outside of India often emphasizes the physical benefits of yoga, many who do hatha yoga are profoundly aware of its mental, spiritual, and emotional benefits. Many of the asanas, or physical yoga poses, assist in strengthening and increasing flexibility in the joints and along the spine. Major chakras lie along the joints of the spine and minor chakras rotate along other axis of the body and places like the hands and feet. Hatha yoga, when done with careful attention to alignment and right intention, can be of benefit to the physical body and assist in energetically clearing the chakras. If you would like to practice hatha yoga and are not doing so, many yoga studios and gyms offer classes with qualified instructors.

The following is a list of chakras and general asanas that assist in opening the chakras.

It is always important to consult a qualified yoga instructor to assist you in practicing yoga.

✦ Muladhara (Root) Chakra. The root chakra's ability to connect the spiritual with the earth element is enhanced by standing poses, especially vigorous poses where the knees are bent like Warrior One and Two or Thunderbolt.

✦ Svadhisthana (Sacral) Chakra. Yoga poses that increase flexibility in the lumbar spine(lower back) and hip joints open the sacral chakra. Sitting cross legged can help open the hips and the emotional energy center, or a bent knee pigeon lunge are some examples. The Bridge pose helps to increase flexibility in the lumbar spine.

✦ Manipura (Belly) Chakra. When in balance the belly chakra bestows authentic power and inner confidence. Abdominal strengthening like Boat pose awaken the belly chakra which would help one take action in the world. An overly active belly chakra may cause us to be overly aggressive. This center can be quieted with relaxing supported poses that physiologically calm the nervous system, which quiet excess activity, like Viparita Karani, where you lie down with a pillow underneath your hips and your legs up the wall.

✦ Anahata (Heart) Chakra. Back bends like the Cobra and Full wheel help to open the spine and the heart chakra. Shoulder opening stretches also assist in opening the heart center. When we carry our physical carriage with an open heart our energetic heart will open, we can access healthy self-love and compassion for others

✦ Vishuddha (Throat) Chakra. Shoulder stand is excellent for stimulating and balancing all physical aspects of the throat chakra, like the neck, thyroid, and upper respiratory system. Seated forward bends, where the neck is in flexion, quiet the throat chakra. Fish pose, a back bend where the neck is in extreme extension, stimulates the throat chakra.

✦ Ajna (Brow) Chakra. The brow chakra benefits from many poses, including some seated forward bends and handstand. The brow and the crown chakra are enlivened and supported by meditation.

✦ Sahasrara (Crown) Chakra. The crown chakra is stimulated by inversions, where one is upside down and the major chakras are placed in reverse order in relationship to the earth, especially headstand, considered the king of asanas.

bija mantra

The bija mantra for the heart chakra is Yam (pronounced YUM).

CHAPTER 8

throat chakra

tHE THROAT CHAKRA, symbolically represented by the color blue and an empty bowl of ether, is known by the Sanskrit word *vishuddha*, which means "purification." The fifth chakra is the chakra of eloquence of human expression. The vishuddha chakra can manifest in music, visual imagery, or classic literature. Insightful media content or soulful self-expression in relationships qualify as examples of the fifth chakra transmission of spiritual information to the material plane. Our spiritual purpose may be to express new mathematical theories or it may be to communicate with great skill to our loved ones.

The vishuddha chakra represents the loftier side of creativity, and to understand the fifth chakra, it helps to discern the difference between the fifth chakra and the second chakra. The creativity of the second chakra may seem more base and infantile; we create babies, poo, and finger paint from the second chakra. Graffiti with a social message would be a fifth-chakra endeavor, while a graffiti tag is definitely a second chakra act of creation. The universe, however, does not place value judgments on types of creative acts. It is just as important that we make a bowel movement as a wonderful poem. We need one to have the other, and like the chakras, they are interconnected.

Ether, an element observed by the *rishis*, or ancient sages, of India, is of a lighter vibration than air and represents the vishuddha chakra. The great spiritual teacher Yogananda used to illustrate the element of ether by telling a story about people who were blind and had their sight miraculously restored. At first the formerly blind individuals would see everything flat. A world without ether would be two-dimensional. Sound, as a vibration, travels through space, and the fifth chakra's symbol is the sixteen-petal lotus flower, each petal corresponding to one of the Sanskrit vowels. A velvet-tongued rapper, an operatic diva, and a fast-talking auctioneer all use the fifth chakra's ability to create sound as a vibration.

The fifth chakra also governs the *yin* side of sound: silence and listening. Someone who talks without listening, interrupts, or talks over his or her conversation partner may be speaking from a place of imposing their power. Rather than listening to the silence between notes, the space between breaths, a fearful or ungrounded person may babble on annoyingly and incessantly. Perhaps self-absorbed and coming from a place like the egotistical third chakra, many fail to master the lesson that listening is just as important as speaking in communication. For true communication occurs in understanding, not dictating. Inconsiderate cell phone man, as the movie commercial shows us, is not using the power of space in his fifth chakra. Instead he blasts open the aperture of his vishuddha center, dictating his communications indiscriminately.

listening practice

Next time you engage in a conversation, notice how many times you feel you need to get a point across. Often our own ideas and ego get in the way of listening. We are so busy trying to say something that we often don't listen. Try to allow an idea to arise that you want to com- municate, see if you can let it go and not talk about it. A friend wants to talk to you about her idea for a short story. You want to tell her about the plot of a similar story you read in a literature course. Instead, keep quiet and notice that the conversation will continue without your every input and that your ability to listen is enhanced as you distance yourself from thoughts that are stimulated in daily dialogs. If you can't listen well, your throat chakra may be blocked. Try avoiding pungent-flavored drinks and foods and caffeine to assist in balancing the vishuddha center.

Technology is playing a big role in facilitating modern communication and as a result is pushing the envelope of our spiritual evolution. Through cell phones, computers, and other electronic devices, we are receiving more information and communication instantaneously. As our material technology evolves, we have the opportunity to use it to rise to new levels of spiritual power or to succumb to information overload. As we climb to the elevated stages of power and consciousness in the three upper chakras, we must use this power responsibly. In the fifth chakra, it is our responsibility to speak our truth from a place of honesty and integrity, even when people who are steeped in illusion are resistant. We may be put in a position where we have no choice but to expose their conscious or unconscious delusions.

The throat chakra also connects to the hand chakras, which is where we manifest symbolically and literally. The refined creative element of the fifth chakra manifests creative works that are expansive and evocative to mankind. The vishuddha chakra also governs telepathic communication. We may hear voices of people who aren't physically present or hear *disincarnate* spirits through the clairaudient channels.

The fifth chakra's glandular association is with the thyroid and the parathyroid. The thyroid secretes the hormone thyroxine, essential to normal body growth, and is also involved in digestion and metabolism. The thyroid is the only organ in the body that actually takes up iodine, and it can make thyroxine only if there is enough organic iodine available through the diet. The parathyroid gland, embedded in the thyroid gland, helps maintain proper calcium levels, which, if raised too high, can lead to kidney stones and kidney failure. The throat chakra is physically related to the throat, neck, and upper respiratory system.

● ● ● butterfly ● ● ●

The shape of the thyroid gland resembles a butterfly, symbolizing elevated transformation. The thyroid will thrive on this alkalizing, mineral-rich juice. Iodine, which the thyroid requires, is found most reliably in sea vegetables and organic produce. However, iodine will only be present in vegetables grown in iodine-rich soil, therefore sea vegetables, such as dulse, provide insurance that iodine is included in the diet. Ginger clears communication and is good for the throat and upper respiratory system. A sulphur compound found in the radish is a regulator of the thyroid hormones, thyroxine, and calcitonin. This recipe is by Lisa Bach of Juicey Lucy's 100% Vegetarian Organic Kosher Café and Juice Bar.

- 2–3 medium apples
- 1-inch cube daikon radish
- 3 lactino (dinosaur) kale leaves
- 3 large collard green leaves
- 1-inch cube ginger, unpeeled
- ¼-inch cube of fennel

After juicing these ingredients, pour into a 16-ounce container. If you have made less than 16 ounces, juice more apples until you have a total of 16 ounces of juice. Stir in ½ teaspoon dulse flakes gently into the juice using a wooden utensil. A chopstick works well. Drinking Butterfly juice will leave you singing with joy.

••• blueberry listening shake •••

A blue shake that is excellent for the thyroid and metabolic process. Coconut water heals the thyroid and parathyroid gland. Blueberries, a sacred food of Native Americans, are now considered by modern science to be a superfood because of their high levels of antioxidant phyto-nutrients. Blueberries help us cultivate the light vibratory frequency of ether symbolized by the color blue. Kids will love this drink, and it could help them develop the ability to hear what the adults are trying to say to them.

- 1–2 cups raw or canned young coconut water (sometimes called juice)
- (optional) ½ cup raw, young coconut meat
- ¼–½ cup blueberries
- ½ cup Heaven and Earth Almond Milk (see recipe page 69)
- 1 date
- **Bonus super ingredient**: 1 tablespoon flaxseed oil (omega-3 efa for thyroid support)

If you take the coconut water from a fresh coconut, you can enrich Blueberry Listening Shake and add EFAs from the coconut meat. Open the young coconut to remove the juice and then scrape the soft meat out of the inside. Place in the blender along with the date, pitted and chopped into small pieces; blueberries; almond milk; and bonus super ingredient. Blend on high speed until smooth, or creamy if you used the coconut meat.

••• talk to me baby •••

This recipe stimulates soulful communication with the ones you love. Coats throat, stimulates liver. Christie McClelland of Gayatri Healing contributed this recipe.

- 1 pint blueberries
- 1 cup purified water
- 1 apple
- 2 teaspoons honey
- 1 lemon

Juice the apple and lemon. Blend with blueberries and honey. Add water to reach the desired consistency. Add ice cubes for a shake.

••• speak easy ether tea •••

Gotu kola is a revered Ayurvedic herb and is known as "the secret of perpetual youth." It is an adaptogen that balances hormones and stimulates the thyroid. Licorice root is sattvic and enhances balance, peace, and harmony in one's life. Marshmallow energizes the throat chakra and is good for coughs. Ginger and lemon are always great for soothing and coating the throat for singing or speaking. Jaggery has cleansing properties, especially effective on the upper respiratory system. Speak Easy Ether Tea will harmonize the throat chakra and add ease, grace, and joy to your communications.

- 1 teaspoon licorice root
- 1 teaspoon marshmallow root
- ½ teaspoon gotu kola
- ¼–½ teaspoon grated ginger
- Juice of ½ lemon
- 2–3 cups purified water
- (optional) 1 tablespoon jaggery or other appropriate sweetener

Place licorice root, marshmallow root, and gotu kola in a tea bag, teapot, or French press. Boil water and pour over the herbs. Steep for 15 minutes. Strain if necessary. Add ginger, lemon juice, and sweetener.

bija mantra

The bija mantra for the throat chakra is Ham (pronounced HUM).

vipassana

Vipassana is one of India's ancient techniques of meditation. Rediscovered by Buddha, who saw it as the remedy for all ills, Vipassana is usually taught in residence. It uses the premise that by observing the breath during prolonged periods of silence to concentrate the mind, one can understand universal truths of impermanence, suffering, and egolessness. Practiced outside the confines of religion, it seeks to impart universal truths through a method that people from all faiths can use. Participants say the silence and noncommunication allows one to detach from the turbulent energies of the lower chakras.

ionized alkaline water

Water ionizers are electrical devices that take low-pH tap water and transform it into water that replicates pure mountain stream water, which is highly alkaline and life- giving. The reason mountain stream water has such wonderful flavor and energy can be explained scientifically. At high altitudes the atmosphere thins, so there is more UV light and cosmic rays. As water bounces off the rocks in the mountains, it picks up hydroxyl ions, making smaller water molecule clusters and creating delicious alkaline water. Water ionizers make water that mimics mountain streams by using a process known as electrolysis; the ionizer adds hydroxyl ions, thereby alkalizing water that has been stripped of its life by chemical process and filtration. Water ionizers were first invented in Japan more than fifty years ago. For many years, ionizers were only used in Japanese hospitals, where they reduced recovery time following surgery by half. Finally a little over a decade ago they were introduced for public use. "Mother nature never intended for us to drink from a tap," says Jim Karnstedt, owner of the Ion and Light Company, which specializes in selling the relatively unknown water ionizers in the United States. In addition, the ionized water "creates smaller water clusters, [and] it hydrates your cells six times as effectively as bottled or tap water," explains Karnstedt. Ionized water can measure up to a 9.5 pH and should not be taken with meals, as it offsets the natural acidity of the stomach necessary for digestion. Because herbs naturally alkalize minerals, adding herbs to water in the form of hot or ice tea is a natural way to make ordinary water more alkaline. Some new designer waters, such as Essentia, are selling ionically separated purified water. Essentia has a pH of 9.5 and is available in most health food stores.

daily fluid intake

To determine your minimum daily fluid intake: Take your weight in pounds, divide this number in half. This number is the minimum number of ounces of noncaffeinated tea or water you should be drinking per day. For example, a person who weighs 150 pounds should drink seventy-five ounces of water daily. For every alcoholic, caffeinated, or carbonated drink you consume, rehydrate your body by drinking the same quantity of water or nonalcoholic or noncaffeinated drink in addition to your daily required fluid intake. For exercise, add eight ounces of water for every fifteen minutes of aerobic activity.

CHAPTER 9

brow chakra

The BROW, or *ajna*, chakra is the center of vision, illumination, and imagination. Its elemental association with light relates to the pineal gland, which itself produces hormones in accord with the body's exposure to natural light. Everyone has an innate ability to visualize. Visual imagery is the language of the spirit and its seat is in the sixth chakra.

The brow chakra is the center of imagination, where our soul creates and deciphers images of the psyche. Shamans use their brow chakra to enter the dreamtime, a deep trance that allows them to connect to a realm beyond the physical communing with the spirits of people, plants, and animals. In the dreamtime, one can time-travel to any place in the past, present, or future. The physical world is paralleled in the dreamtime, yet it exists outside of the constraints of time, like our sleeping dreams.

As we climb up through the chakras, the sixth chakra elucidates truth and creates visions that can transform our lives, living up to the meaning of ajna: authority, command, unlimited power. When comparing the chakras to the tree of life, the sixth and seventh chakras are like a foundation or seed, which will grow into physical manifestation. They are like the roots of the tree in the kabalistic model, which originate in the spiritual and grow out into physical manifestation. The creative process begins with a vision from the brow or crown chakra and then is brought to the earth through the root chakra. In the kabala, or tree of life, it is the base of the tree that is thought and the top of the tree is the earth, where visions manifest. In this way the circle of creation is represented in the chakras, as the base becomes the brow and crown chakras, which create what happens on the earth plane in the root chakra.

anyone can visualize

Close your eyes and see in your mind's eye your bed and your bedroom. You can do this from any location. You can also lie in your bed and see the bedroom as though you were viewing it through your eyes as you lay on the bed or you can see yourself in the bed, like in a movie. The important thing is realizing you are seeing without the physical use of your eyes. On an energetic level, this very simply is what the third eye does. Knowing that you can visualize may empower you to practice visualization.

Another way to practice with your third eye is to observe people you find interesting with your physical eyes.

Notice how ideas about these people come to you through your imagination. You see with your physical eyes and then move to a deeper level, where your brow chakra and your intuition kicks in. It is easier to use clairvoyance or intuition on total strangers because without preconceived notions or emotional investments you can access pure observation and intuition more easily.

At the level of the ajna chakra there is no comparing mind, but simply the discernment of light and dark. We need the fire of our ego to act, but we need the intuition of our sixth chakra to know how to act from our personal truth. The late, Yogi Bhajan, founder of Kundalini yoga, taught that the only true security is available through our intuition. If we seek to satisfy our ego, our third eye will remain closed. Yogi Bhajan says that when we give up our ego, a void is created, and into this void our intuition will be drawn. He advises that when we practice silence daily, we cultivate our intuitive powers. Buddhists have long been connoisseurs of silence who allow a higher power to reveal itself in quiet moments. Thus the security of the body and the lower chakras is fed by our intuition, which is a deeper, more foundational security. When we don't listen to our intuition, our body will act out like a child through stress, fear, and anger. Our emotions will also possibly block our clairvoyance as we become emotionally attached to people or outcomes of certain situations.

Many people want to use clairvoyance, yet the truth quite often shatters the illusions most would prefer to keep it at bay. Often the "crazy" people in our society experience sudden clairvoyant or revelatory openings and have no idea how to integrate their visions into ordinary life. Without a strong earth connection, the hallucinatory visions of the ajna chakra can leave one in a disassociated mental state. Of course, it is possible to look through the third eye and remain sane. It just requires the ability to see the greater lesson in all of people's difficulties and challenges. Clairvoyance is the challenging and piercing ability to see the truth. We all have an innate ability to use our third eye and pierce the veil of physical reality, but do we really want to know the truth?

meditation

Dharana is concentration of the mind. Visualize and place your attention on each of the seven major chakras individually, using color and location in the body. Spend one to five minutes on each one, focusing the mind and allowing whatever arises into consciousness to emerge. This meditation will have two benefits; one is focusing the mind and the other is uncovering personal experiential knowledge of the chakras.

••• **mystic mango smoothie** •••

The mango is considered the king of fruits in Ayurveda. It is rich in bioflavonoids, antioxidants, potassium, fiber, and vitamin C. This light fruit shake activates the vibration of light in the upper chakras; combined with the fanciful influence of blackberries, you will attain a sublime mind. Add the adaptogen royal jelly, which powers up the pineal and pituitary glands, and your center of light will be buzzing with a delectable whirl of vibrant antioxidants and universal life force. This one is great for kids too, but don't add royal jelly or bonus ingredients!

- ¾ cup fresh (preferably) or frozen blackberries
- 1 mango, pitted and chopped (note that imported mangos that are not organic are often sprayed with chemicals banned in the United States.)
- ¼–½ cup purified water
- 1 tablespoon flaxseed oil
- 1 small vial royal jelly (.33 ounces or 1 tablespoon)
- **Bonus super ingredients:** 1 teaspoon maca powder or 1 teaspoon ashwagandha, both for a pituitary and pineal gland boost, hormonal support, and stress buffers; ¼–⅛ teaspoon Etherium Gold (see sidebar on monatomic minerals).

Place ingredients in a blender, blend, and serve.

monatomic minerals

Monatomic minerals are believed to affect our chakras and energy bodies and in powder form can be added to smoothies and other chakra tonics. Physicists call monatomic minerals exotic matter because they have exceptional antigravitational and superconductive abilities. A company called Harmonic Innerprizes sells naturally occurring monatomic minerals that were discovered in the Shasta Mountains in California and are safe for human consumption. The company's founder Pat Bailey became interested in monatomic minerals came after hearing a lecture by David Hudson, a leading researcher on the subject.

Working in the supplements industry for more than twenty years, Bailey founded Rainbow Light, the first company to produce whole foods-based vitamins. Pursuing a lifelong passion for study and investigation into health and energy medicine, he personally formulated the health food industry's bestselling cold and flu remedy, Source Naturals' Wellness Formula. When he heard stories of a Choctaw healer who was having amazing results curing cancer and AIDS with an herb called chamae rose, which was not known at the time for its medicinal properties, he paid her a visit. Bailey followed a hunch that the miracle cures were not because of the plant she used but instead a result of the soil where the plant grew. He took a sample and began his research. He sent the claylike white powder to a regular lab, which found nothing.

Next he tried analysis by another lab that specialized in measuring the electromagnetic field surrounding materials and had a history of testing earth samples from the world's top mines. The second lab's president was dumbfounded when the material's frequencies appeared on paper as if they were a diagram from a physics textbook, showing the configuration of energy turning into matter. The lab's president told Bailey he believed the soil was so powerful that it had the potential to regenerate life on earth. At the same time Bailey had pills made from the powder and passed them out to friends, who reported increased creativity and enhanced meditation practices.

One of the friends brought sample capsules to a well-known Los Angeles medium, who channels an entity named Bashar, to inquire about their potency. Bashar told him, "Sir, the capsules that you have in your hand are beyond your comprehension of electromagnetic properties. The capsules that you have in your hand can best be described as electromagnatheria, those being substances that are being brought forth in your space-time reality to help the human vibration become more at one, more aligned with the Universal vibrations that surround you. As a result, it is given to you at this time as a gift from the Ascended Masters who are guiding the destiny of your planet into the New Age, which you all purport to be a part of."

Bashar thus psychically validated the accuracy of the lab's electromagnetic analysis and created a demand among his devotees for this high-frequency dirt. And so Bailey began his new business, Harmonic Innerprizes. These monatomic minerals are naturally occurring and were found where a meteorite was believed by scientists to have hit the earth around 11,000 years ago somewhere in the Shasta Mountains of California. These products come in pill or powder form. The powder can be added to smoothies or taken under the tongue.

Etherium Gold's benefits have since been investigated in several bona fide clinical scientific studies. One study concluded through EEG analysis that Etherium Gold helps increase both theta (right brain) and beta(left brain) waves and balance both wave frequencies, therefore helping individuals become more whole brained. Etherium Gold stimulates the upper chakras, especially the brow and the crown chakra, increasing creativity and enhancing meditation practice.

Etherium Pink, another one of Harmonic Innerprizes' products, helps to heal and balance emotions and especially the heart chakra. It assists in attaining clarity in our emotions by opening the heart chakra, which in turn increases our capacity for compassion for others and opens up potential for self acceptance and understanding.

Etherium Red stimulates Kundalini energy, which originates in the root chakra and then travels up the sushuma nadi to cleanse and heal all seven bodily chakras. Etherium Red vibrates the throat chakra, the hormonal system, and the thyroid. The MHz frequencies in Harmonic Innerprizes Red are comparable with the frequencies that are inherent in the glands that comprise the endocrine system, especially the thyroid.

Etherium Black helps to release any negative spiritual energy that has come to affect our physical bodies. It has become a favorite remedy for people who have consumed too much alcohol as a hangover cure. Etherium Black is also used extensively by massage therapists and other healers who want to clear the energy they absorb in giving healings, especially to extremely ill or disturbed individuals. Etherium Black also helps to dispel allergies and allergic reactions.

All Etherium products are sold as Supplements for the Spirit and can be purchased online at :
www.harmonicinnerprizes.com.

. . . .

... **third eye tonic** ...

This tonic balances intuition and intellect. The pomegranate looks like a red or earthy brain; the chamomile flowers relax and open the lower chakras and the third eye. Pomegranates are now being marketed heavily for their antioxidant properties. Don't forget their terrific ability to ground the brain and stimulate creative and innovative thought. It's a much needed quality in our society, so its no wonder pom juice is all the rage!

- 1 pomegranate or 1–½ cup prepared pomegranate juice
- 8 ounces purified water
- 1 teaspoon chamomile flowers or 1 chamomile tea bag
- 1 cinnamon stick
- 5 cloves

Boil the water and steep the chamomile, cinnamon, and cloves in it. Break the pomegranate into 4–8 pieces and juice (or use 1½ cups pre-made pomegranate juice). Allow to cool or mix warm with the pomegranate juice. Add sweetener if desired.

••• meditation lemonade •••

Meditation calms the mind and has an alkalinizing affect on our water bodies. However, if we are in an acidic state, the mind is rampant with mental chatter, making meditation a challenging feat. Meditation Lemonade will help alkalize the body's pH, making it less difficult to sit. You will fidget less and feel refreshed. Watermelon is a highly alkaline fruit, while whispers of lemongrass invoke the wisdom of the ajna chakra. Fresh lemons, although acidic, have an overall alkalinizing effect on the body.

- 4 cups watermelon cut in chunks
- 4 cups lemongrass tea
- Juice of 5 lemons
- 2 tablespoons to ¼ cup agave or 1 tablespoon stevia to taste

Make lemongrass tea with 2–4 lemongrass tea bags and four cups of boiling water. To make lemongrass tea with fresh lemongrass, take 2–3 stalks of lemongrass and cut into 3-inch pieces. Place in a saucepan and with 4½ cups of purified water, bring to a boil, and then simmer 5–10 minutes. Allow tea to cool. Place in a blender with other ingredients, blend, and voila. Your mind is at peace as you sip this delicious elixir.

••• peek-a-boo •••

This juice will do wonders for your physical eyesight, directly related to the third eye. When outer vision is cloudy, so sometimes is inner vision. Orange bell peppers offer the richest source of zeaxanthin, which along with lutein prevents age-related macular degeneration and a host of other eye problems. Some have even called the carotenoids in leafy greens and orange bell peppers sunglasses for the eyes.

- 2 dinosaur kale leaves
- 2 dandelion leaves
- 1 orange bell pepper
- 5 carrots

Juice these ingredients and stir! You will alkalize your body and heal outer/inner vision with Peek-a-Boo!

••• cosmic wisdom tea •••

The upper chakras respond well to many herbal teas, especially floral, fragrant, and bitter blends. Cosmic Wisdom Tea visually and energetically represents the enlightened wisdom of the ajna chakra. Red clover, a sacred medicinal herb of European culture, was believed to represent the Trinity. The plant's leaves are the inspiration for the suit of clubs in ordinary playing cards. Chamomile, a favorite tea, brings in the holy golden wisdom of a greater power as it soothes and relaxes nervous tension. Jasmine flowers are said to carry psychic frequencies to the physical realm and make the mind more receptive to them. In the Ayurvedic tradition, jasmine flowers resonate in accord and assist the power of mantras.

- 1 teaspoon clover flowers
- 1½ teaspoon chamomile flowers
- ½ teaspoon jasmine flowers
- 2–3 cups purified water

Place flower blend in a French press or individual tea bag, cup, or teapot. Pour boiling water over the blend; steep for 15 minutes, strain if necessary. Serve with honey or other appropriate sweetener.

neti pot

One of a group of six actions of purification of body and mind, *neti* has a direct and significant action of opening the third eye. The other five actions cleanse the lower chakras, except *trataka*, a practice of gazing at a candle or other object until the eyes tear. Traditionally neti is performed with a long-beaked pot called a *loka*. Warm water is mixed with a small amount of salt and the solution is poured from the loka through one nostril as the practitioner leans forward bending at the waist until the nostril in which the salt water is entering is higher than the other nostril. The saline wash exits through the opposite nostril. The neti is very invigorating, cleansing to the nasal passages, and helpful in preventing colds and flu before they occur. Benefits of this ancient Indian practice were discovered in a Wake Forest University study where thirty patients who used a saline nasal wash showed significant decreased allergic inflammation. Other studies have shown increased immune response in those participating in nasal irrigation. Many practitioners who perform a daily nasal wash report increased mental clarity and an opening of the energetic channels of clairvoyance in the ajna chakra or third eye.

... krishna tulsi tea with honey ...

Tulsi, or royal basil, sacred to Vishnu and Krishna, promotes the energy of attachment and is said to be a sacred elixir. Tulsi means "the incomparable one." A majestic herb that Ganesh wears in a sacred garland around his neck, tulsi is similar to, but different from, Italian basil. Both can be used for tea or healing purposes. Having a basil plant in your home is said to purify the air and clear negative frequencies from the home. Next to lotus, holy basil is the most sacred plant in India, traditionally used to open the heart and mind. In India there are many types of tulsi, Krishna tulsi is purple, the color of the brow chakra, and is believed by some to be the most powerful tulsi. Other common Indian basils are *rama* and *vana* tulsi. Tulsi tea with honey is pure sattva and is a drink recommended in Ayurveda for all people. The health benefits of royal basil are being confirmed by scientific research; tulsi is a premier adaptogen, supporting the heart, lungs, and liver, among other organs. Tulsi has antiaging properties, antiviral, antifungal, antioxidant, and anti-inflammatory properties, and it is known to reduce side effects associated with allopathic medicine. Tulsi, in fact, has hundreds of life-enhancing properties and is known to be one of the eight things indispensable to Vedic worship. Tulsi tea delivers nutrients necessary for enlightenment. In addition to tulsi's lessening the negative spiritual vibrations of everyday stressors, its use will attract excellent overall health, and cultivate peace, joy, and states of higher awareness. Dried Krishna tulsi or a mixture of

Krishna, Rama, and Vana Tulsi, is available in bulk from Organic India, *www.organicindiausa.com.*

- 2–3 cups boiled purified water
- 2–3 teaspoons dried Krishna tulsi (or a blend of Krishna, Rama, and Vana Tulsi)
- 1–2 teaspoons raw honey or other appropriate sweetener
- 1–3 crushed fresh basil leaves
- (optional) 1 cinnamon stick

Boil water; add Krishna tulsi in an infuser or tea bag along with fresh basil (from your garden or the market, fresh basil will supercharge the life energy in this tea) and optional cinnamon stick. Steep for 5–10 minutes. Add honey and enjoy daily!

bija mantra

The brow chakra's bija mantra is Om (pronounced AUM). This is one of the most chanted syllables on the planet. This sound represents divine presence and will invoke higher levels of consciousness when chanted vibrantly.

tulsi tea collection

B rewing homemade tea blends can seem complicated and time consuming if you lead a busy life. If you are not inclined to make your own teas, try keeping it simple. Buy a bunch of fresh mint and brew your own tisane with it or get a potted rosemary plant that you can use to make fresh tea or use as a seasoning. If you are inclined to use only store-bought tea bags, I highly recommend Organic India Tulsi Tea line. These high-quality teas are made with holy basil, also known as tulsi. Organic India is an ecological and spiritually minded company that makes wonderful teas that can be used to tune and open the chakras and heal the body. Tulsi is in every blend and helps boost immunity, relieve stress, increase stamina, and promotes a healthy metabolism without any harmful side effects. Tulsi has natural antioxidant, antibacterial, antiviral, and adaptogenic properties. It's a sacred herb recommended for those on a spiritual path.

Tulsi Ginger. This blend will help to ground and stimulate digestion. It works well as an overall tonic.

Tulsi Chai. This blend has a lot of fire and will help stimulate energy and the belly chakra. It contains caffeine.

Tulsi Darjeeling. This blend has tulsi and Darjeeling, which contains caffeine and will energize the body, mind, and spirit. Don't use this tea if you already feel overstimulated.

Tulsi Green Tea. This delicious combo will energize and open the upper chakras. Although slightly stimulating, due to the caffeine content of green tea, this tea is a good all-around chakra tonic.

Tulsi Gotu Kola. This combo will open your upper chakras and connect you to cosmic wisdom and transcendent thought patterns. This would be a good blend if you need to do a lot of creative thinking, studying, or meditating.

Tulsi teas, by Organic India, are available in many health food stores or online at: *www.organicindiausa.com.*

••• heavy metal banned •••

Due to increasing environmental pollution, our brains and bodies may be exposed to harmful levels of heavy metals. Overexposure causes oxidative stress and is associated with the development of neurodegenerative diseases. One meta-analysis found that cadmium, aluminum, and mercury are present at much higher levels in people diagnosed with Alzheimer's disease. How can you fight back? Drink Heavy Metal Banned to detoxify the brain and release the burden of environmental pollutants. This tangy juice packs a powerful punch of antioxidants and chelation factors that will help your organs and gut detox daily whenever you imbibe this delicious juice. Use this tonic to expand your third eye to access the clear seeing, or clairvoyance, of a balanced ajna center. (Known as ajna, or command center, the brow chakra is associated with the brain.) Reducing the toxic burden of environmental pollution is critical to all levels of spiritual, emotional, and physical health. This juice decreases brain fog and promotes clarity of vision.

- 3 organic apples (sweet variety), use 4 if you like it sweeter
- 1 organic Meyer lemon
- ½–1 organic lime
- ½ cup loosely packed and barely chopped organic cilantro
- 7.5 mg of chlorella tincture without alcohol, or ½ teaspoon of chlorella powder

Cut the apples in quarters, then core them and remove the seeds. Cut the Meyer lemon and lime and remove the seeds. Using a juicer, extract the juice from the apples, Meyer lemon, and lime. Wash and loosely cut the cilantro so it will fit in a measuring cup. Then add the fresh juice, cilantro, and chlorella into a blender. Blend until the tonic has a silky texture and a beautiful green color.

••• self-actualization smoothie •••

Prepare this smoothie as you contemplate becoming the best version of yourself. According to Maslow's theory of self-actualization, fulfilling one's potential is a drive found in everyone. It's not about improvement, but aligning yourself with your true nature: the most powerful and magnetic version of you. When we are self-actualized, we feel our hearts, minds, and divine connections working togeth-

er. The journey of self-actualization has many challenges, but the
rewards are priceless. This smoothie helps you to build stamina
and sharpen the mind. Our integrity and consciousness help us to
use our knowledge for good. Tahini contains the brain-boosting
phenolic compound sesamol. Tahini also is high in Omega-3 fats,
which are anti-inflammatory and have been shown to lower risk of
neurodegenerative diseases. As a remedy, spirulina is extraordinary;
it's anti-inflammatory, antioxidant, immune enhancing, and neuro-
protective properties have efficacy comparable to a pharmaceutical
drug according to the scientific literature.

- 1 cup unsweetened almond milk (make your own by
  following the recipe for Heaven on Earth Almond Milk
  on pages 69-70)
- 2 dates, pitted
- ¼ cup tahini
- ½ teaspoon powdered spirulina
- ½ teaspoon cardamom powder
- ½ teaspoon ginger powder

Pour the almond milk into a blender. Pit and chop the dates into
a few pieces, and add the tahini, spirulina, cardamom, and ginger.
Blend until smooth. Drink and enjoy.

CHAPTER 10

crown chakra

I cured with the power that came through me. Of course it was not I who cured, it was the power from the Outer World, the visions and the ceremonies had only made me like a hole through which power could come through two-leggeds.

—BLACK ELK

"I KNEW IT off the top of my head" is an expression that explicates the crown chakra's ability to bring in information from the cosmos. Covering the crown like an invisible cap, the *sahasrara* chakra governs thoughts and symbolizes the guru within, or *upa* guru. Our thoughts create our world. Thought, sahasrara's element, moves faster than the element of light in the sixth chakra. If we are going to climb a mountain, we need the sound health that comes with harmony in the lower chakras, yet we also need the belief or inspiration that we can climb up the mountain. An ill or physically weak person may be able to will themselves up the mountain with their thoughts. A physically fit person may not be able to control their thoughts and may get distracted from climbing the mountain. As we begin to observe and control our thoughts, we realize their power.

Our thoughts, broadcast from the thousand-petal lotus flower that is the crown, create our universe. When we gain mastery over the volatile and speedy power of our thoughts, we can link their power to the lower chakras and obtain all *sidhis*, or powers. The yogi who reaches this level is said to meet the *Kamadhenu*, or the wish-fulfilling cow within himself. The crown can become unstable if the turbulent vibrations of the lower chakras are not mastered. Thoughts move at a rapid speed that most people who do not meditate never contemplate or understand. They are, in a sense, prisoners of their thoughts, which often are not even their own.

The crown chakra can act as a doorway, allowing dynamic energy from the cosmos, other entities, or other people to enter and take over. Many call this ability channeling or trance mediumship. The crown is a portal for exit and entry of the physical body. When a person has an open, receptive sahasrara chakra, it operates somewhat like a radio antenna picking up transmissions from the cosmos. This ability can be helpful in seeking celestial guidance, but when unchecked creates inconsistent and erratic behavior. A person with a wide-open crown chakra is a bit like a person who has a radio with a broken dial. The broadcast keeps switching from station to station, unable to commit to one particular frequency. The lack of ability to control the sahasrara crown portal can create minor inconsistencies in personalities or, in severe cases, schizophrenia.

You may loan your car to someone who appears responsible and alert and then crashes into five cars. You may have a bizarre relative who changes his opinion from one day to the next, a daydreaming coworker, or a spouse who always forgets to pay the bills. All of these examples are of people, often extremely creative and industrious, who have difficulty in anchoring their capabilities to the dense earthly vibration. These people are like radios that can't tune in to a particular station so they keep switching stations, lacking consistency. Unable to harness their overwhelming power, these personality types are often brimming with ideas but have trouble carrying out their plans. Teenagers are unusually quick to display the frequent channel shifting of the crown chakra; most do not know themselves well enough to commit to the unwavering command needed to steer the thousand-pedaled lotus of the crown chakra.

The seventh chakra is where we ascend from our earthly body when we die, and therefore the seventh chakra is the chakra of immortality or ascension. As Kundalini energy travels up the chakras, individuality is transcended in the sahasrara chakra. When one is able to integrate all of the seven major chakras, a kind of heaven on earth may be experienced in which one realizes the divinity within oneself. Teachers and great leaders communicate from this chakra and use it to broadcast their message, spiritually as well as vocally. The seventh chakra governs the pituitary gland, the master gland, and in some traditions the sahasrara vibrates at such a high frequency that it cannot be associated with physical processes. Children will respond better when you speak to their soul essence. Through this chakra all of our higher selves are connected.

••• vision quest tea •••

Gotu kola has a long tradition as a tea for yogis and meditators, who drink it to inspire awakening in the sahasrara chakra. Skullcap promotes heightened perception. Mint provides a flavor and a sattvic quality to the blend. Drink Vision Quest Tea for new inspiration from the cosmos or to increase your aptitude for meditation.

- 1 teaspoon mint
- 1 teaspoon skullcap
- 1 teaspoon gotu kola
- 3 cups purified water

Place herbs in a French press, teapot, or tea bag. Steep in boiling water and enjoy.

••• lemon-barley water •••

Recipes for barley water can be found everywhere from Ayurvedic cookbooks to gourmet websites. Barley is considered a sacred grain, and long before Sprite, people served lemon-barley water regularly. It's yummy and good for you. Barley water is an excellent cleanser for the kidneys and teamed with lemon makes a wonderful healing beverage that is delicious warm or cool.

- ¼ cup organic pearl barley
- 3 ½–4 cups purified water
- 1 lemon
- 1–2 tablespoons of agave or suitable sweetener
- 1 handful of fresh cranberries, when in season

Rinse the pearl barley, then place in the water with the cranberries (optional). Simmer for at least ½ hour or until there is a little more than 1 cup of liquid. Juice the lemon and grate the zest. Add lemon juice and zest to the hot water and barley. Steep for 1 or 2 more minutes. Strain, add sweetener, and enjoy.

Lemon-Barley Water makes a highly alkalizing party drink, worthy of a high-energy chakra tonic soiree. Use the following measurements for a party-size batch.

- 2 cups organic pearl barley
- 8 quarts purified water (2 gallons)
- Zest and juice of 8–12 lemons
- ½–1 cup agave or other sweetener

walking meditation

As your energy evolves through the levels of the chakras, the importance of meditation increases, but many on-the-go Westerners have great difficulty sitting in silence. Some great alternatives to silent meditation are walking, knitting, or even driving. These activities will bring about a meditative mental state as the unconscious mind engages in the task of knitting, steering, or pacing.

Try a walking meditation to access the benefits of the sahasrara chakra. Walking engages the subconscious and quiets the turbulent fluctuations of the mind that arise from the lower chakras. It alleviates stress and alkalizes the body.

Walk in silence in the early morning or evening between six and seven pm. Observe your thoughts during your stroll. Notice how your mind slows and you can focus your mind more clearly.

••• angel's realm •••

When we get stuck in the worries and difficulties of the dense earthly plane, angels remind us of the lightness of life. When you integrate the wisdom of the sahasrara chakra you will create a union of the root chakra with the enlightenment of angels. The luminous, white daikon radish represents this journey to transcendence. Its shape resembles the path of Kundalini, traveling up the sushuma nadi to the white/violet portal of transcendence, or crown chakra. Purple cabbage provides a violet note in this symphony of vegetation. Angel's Realm connects you with the power of your inner deity. Lisa Bach of Juicey Lucy's 100% Organic Kosher Café and Juice Bar contributed this recipe!

Juice the following in order to make 16 ounces of juice:

- 2–3 Apples (preferably Fuji or other sweet variety)
- ⅛ of a purple cabbage
- ¼ of a of golden beet
- 1-inch cube of daikon radish
- 1-inch cube of ginger

Pour juice into a 16-ounce container, if you have less than 16 ounces, juice more apples until you have filled a 16-ounce glass or pitcher.

••• seventh chakra divine elixir •••

This light, sweet drink will connect you to your higher self. Chef Christie McClelland, of Gayatri Healing, contributed this recipe.

- 1 pint blackberries
- 2 cups purified water
- 2 tablespoons honey
- 4 oranges or tangerines

Blend and enjoy. For less thickness add more water.

bija mantra

The sound of the crown chakra is silence. As Sanskrit scholar Jay Deva Kumar writes, "All the colors of the rainbow make pure white. All sounds are the manifestation of cosmic silence."

••• mystic mint and lavender tea •••

This tea is intended to expand your connection to the divine, sooth your nervous system, and relax your body. This delicious tea is best enjoyed before bed or between two and six o'clock in the evening when, according to Ayurveda, the subtle energy of ether or space becomes more activated. Additionally, Mystic Mint and Lavender Tea pairs well with the crown chakra ritual on page 183.

- 5–8 fresh spearmint leaves or 1 teaspoon of dried peppermint or spearmint leaves
- ½ teaspoon dried lavender flowers

Place dried herbs in a tea bag or tea ball. If using fresh mint, use a tea press or remove leaves before drinking. Steep for 5 to 7 minutes, then strain. Steep longer if you enjoy strong flavors.

••• cloud 9 astral travel tea •••

Fall asleep quickly with chamomile, a traditional sleep-inducing herb. Its compounds work similarly to sedatives and bind to GABA receptors in the brain. Oat milk has a soothing quality and pairs well with antioxidant rich vanilla powder. Manuka honey has antioxidant and anti-viral properties. Every night you have a powerful opportunity to travel to other dimensions and states of consciousness. You may not think that you are an astral traveler; however, in many cultures, dreaming is a means to go places and do things for healing, understanding, and growth. Sip Cloud 9 Astral Travel Tea so your nighttime itinerary supports your daily life.

- 1 heaping teaspoon of chamomile flowers
- Unsweetened oat milk
- 1 teaspoon vanilla bean powder
- Optional: honey (local honey for allergies or Manuka Honey for immunity)

Fill teacup or mug with unsweetened oat milk.

Prepare a chamomile tea bag or tea ball with the chamomile flowers.

Add the measured milk to a pan and heat on the stove until simmering.

Pour the hot milk back into your mug. Put the tea bag or tea ball into the hot oat milk for about 7 minutes, remove the tea bag or ball, and stir in the vanilla bean powder and honey. Drink and enjoy your dreams.

CHAPTER 11

eighth chakra and the hands and feet chakras

---

tHE EIGHTH CHAKRA, an "out of body" chakra, appears like a halo, and those who have activated this chakra are beings of a certain level of enlightenment. In the past, saints, angels, and avatars all utilized the omnipotent power of the eighth chakra to connect with transcendent forces in the universe. The activation of this chakra will become increasingly possible for ordinary mortals in the future. Make sure you are grounded (see Tree Grounding Visualization, page 167) before you drink any eighth chakra tea.

••• revelation tea •••

Wintergreen is a plant that bears white flowers and is native to the United States. Native Americans long have chewed wintergreen leaves and made tea with this plant, which contains salicylate, chemically related to acetylsalicylic acid, known as modern-day aspirin.

Lavender's pale purple color and lovely calming scent have long been used to connect to transcendent knowledge.

- 2 teaspoons wintergreen leaves
- 1 teaspoon dried lavender flowers, (or 2 teaspoons fresh)
- 3 cups purified water

Place herbs in a French press, teapot, or tea bag. Boil water and pour over blend. Strain if necessary. Serve with raw honey and lemon. A tea for aspiring spiritual leaders and avatars.

hand chakras

The hand chakras are located in the palms and are slightly smaller in circumference than the seven major chakras along the spine. Connected primarily to the heart chakra, the hands also have minor connections to the throat and brow chakras. The hand chakras filter and release our spiritual healing energy. A massage therapist, a painter, and an expert quilt maker will all have developed the database and output of the hand chakras. Fine motor skills, as any child development specialist will tell you, are intimately connected to brain development.

An ability called psychometry, held in the hand chakras, allows one to receive information through touching inanimate objects or people. The hand chakras can channel powerful healing frequencies, such as those used in Reiki therapy. Many cultures have had shamans or healers who must penetrate and reach into the physical body to pull out energies that are not resonating in accord with the physical body. The Philippines and Brazil have long histories of psychic surgeons, or energy healers, who demonstrate this dramatic ability, reaching into a person's body and pulling out what looks like diseased tissue. Many refute these showy "healings" as quackery, yet anthropological investigation reveals similar practices in many cultures throughout recorded history. The Western mind has difficulty grasping this unusual ability of the hand chakras to channel such powerful forces that can cut through physical boundaries.

One woman who has a mission to change our mind-body-spirit patterning through our hands is Vimala Rodgers, whose self-professed goal is to change the world with healthy handwriting. Her website *www.iihs.com* will provide information on how to study and integrate her methods of spiritual penmanship and mastery in the hand chakras.

••• healing hands •••

Rich in minerals, Healing hands is good for fingernails, circulation, and energetic balance. This is a great tea for people who use their hands extensively in their life's work, those who work long hours on computers, or those who are afraid to make things with their hands and have judgment about their handwriting or artwork. Computer work often creates blockages in the hand chakras because the hands absorb electromagnetic energy. On a physical level, this can manifest in carpal tunnel syndrome. Fragrant lemon verbena helps release electromagnetic frequencies and nettles, oatstraw, and horsetail contain important minerals that support the hands and nails. Enjoy your hands. Paint, draw or do some homework. Enjoy.

- 1 teaspoon nettles
- ½ teaspoon horsetail
- ½ teaspoon oat straw
- 2–3 teaspoons fresh lemon verbena or 1½ teaspoons dried
- 3 cups purified water

Place herbs in a French press, teapot, or tea bag. Boil water. Steep until fragrant and enjoy.

feet chakras

Located in the arches of the feet, the feet chakras are connected to the root chakra. The feet chakras assist us in connecting to the earth as we walk upright in the world. Our feet for the most part in the Western world are hidden away in shoes. Ask your average American to remove their shoes at the door and you will get a surprised look.

••• body and sole •••

The soles of the feet receive emanations from the earth. Receiving these important transmissions from the earth was a common practice among Native American tribes who danced the planet's rhythms to connect to Gaia, or Mother Earth. Earth-grown fruits and vegetables dance together in Body and Sole in a refreshing beat that opens and clears the feet chakras.

- 1 sweet potato
- 1 cucumber
- 1 carrot
- ½ fennel bulb (remove stems and save for tea)
- 2 apples

Juice the above ingredients and get your shoes off and your groove on! This juice will have you stomping your feet in celebration! Drink it before dancing!

CHAPTER 12

morning tonics

t HE MORNING is a most auspicious time to drink cleansing tonics; start your day with one of these simple, inexpensive, purifying morning cocktails.

••• new age hot toddy •••

A popular cocktail with the brandy subtracted for the cleansing crowd. The cayenne in this drink makes for a great liver cleanser for those who want a new way to indulge themselves. This recipe was contributed by Christie McClelland of Gayatri Healing.

- ½ lemon
- pinch of cayenne pepper
- 1 teaspoon of raw honey
- ½- to 1-inch chunk ginger

Pour hot water over all and let steep for a while. Drink. Enjoy.

••• **regularity rocks** •••

An alkalizing cleanser to drink upon arising, you will feel 100 percent better balancing your acidic morning cup of tea or coffee with this beverage that tips the acid/alkaline balance back in the right direction. A true natural fiber, psyllium, or plantain seeds, may lower cholesterol according to some studies. They also stimulate and cleanse the intestinal tract, allowing the *apana vayu*, or downward prana, to move freely. Cider vinegar is a natural alkalizer.

- 1 ½ teaspoons organic apple cider vinegar
- 1 teaspoon agave or raw honey
- 1 teaspoon psyllium seed
- 8–12 ounces purified water

Like a martini, serve shaken not stirred. Drink quickly or shake between sips so that those psyllium seeds don't sink to the bottom of the glass.

••• **mnemonic tonic** •••

Rosemary is known as the herb of remembrance; ginkgo biloba is believed to assist in preventing short- and long-term memory loss. Gotu kola balances the right and left sides of the brain. A great tea for those who have a lot to remember or have age-related brain fog!

- 1 teaspoon dried ginkgo biloba leaves
- 1 teaspoon dried gotu kola leaves
- 1 teaspoon dried rosemary (or 1 ½ teaspoons fresh)

Pour hot water over all and let steep for a while. Serve with honey and lemon wedges, this tea has a pungent flavor!

••• morning chant •••

Because Sanskrit is a language of sacred human consciousness, chanting in Sanskrit connects you to divine power. Cranberry's bitter flavor destroys illusions and balances the upper chakras, and a sweet sparkle of tangerine and the powerful immune-enhancing properties of spirulina means that Morning Chant will inspire your day.

- 2 cups cranberries
- 2–3 oranges (or 2 apples)
- 1 heaping teaspoon spirulina

If cranberries are out of season, use ¾ cup unsweetened cranberry juice (Knudsen's Just Cranberry is great!). Use apples if oranges are too acidic for you in the morning. Spirulina is a natural heart opener and cleanser. Stir together ingredients and start singing.

••• grounding future shake •••

The future is now! This heavier tonic integrates and strengthens the lower three chakras, known collectively as the *kanda*, the threefold bulb or seat of fire. As time and technology speed up the vibration of the planet, now more than ever we need to remain grounded, and some of us, but not all, need more protein. According to Julia Ross, author of *The Mood Cure*, diets high in refined carbohydrates wreak havoc on our brains. The convenience foods that were popular and adequate enough for the second half of the twentieth century do not work on our presently overtaxed bodies. If we don't supply our bodies with adequate protein or fats, our mental circuitry fizzles out. We are subject to mood swings, sometimes depression and even manic episodes. This hearty beverage connects us energetically to the worldly plane, synchronizing the spinning of the lower three chakras, and helps us find new enthusiasm in being connected to the earth while we relish in newfound soul awareness. It will go great with the tree visualization.

- 1 cup organic yogurt
- 2 tablespoons almond butter
- ½–1 cup purified water
- ¼ teaspoon finely chopped ginger

Add all ingredients in a blender, blend, and enjoy.

••• fire extinguisher •••

In Ayurveda, diarrhea is caused by an excess of *pitta,* the fire element. The fire element may be activated to eliminate toxins from the body; however, diarrhea can be uncomfortable and cause rapid dehydration. Coconut milk is said to be the world's safest natural soft drink and a natural stress buster according to Ayurveda.

- Juice of one young coconut
- Pinch of nutmeg

Take this tonic as an alternative to Kaopectate. It will not cause constipation.

tree grounding visualization

Visualize that the tip of your tailbone is connected to your favorite tree, one that shades your backyard, one that sheds leaves in the park you frequent, one you remember from your childhood. In your mind's eye, see the oak, redwood, or bodhi tree growing roots into the center of the earth. Connect the trunk to your tailbone and the roots into the center of the earth. Allow the tree to connect you ener- getically to the planet and allow the tree to assist you in releasing any subtle energy that is interfering with your sur- vival and/or your prosperity. Your body is a channel for uni- versal life-force energy. The tree grounding will automatically be connected to all of the chakras through the sushuma nadi, or main energetic channel that runs along the line of the spine, allowing life force that does not belong to you from any chakra to be released into the center of the earth where energy is composted.

Trees connect into the earth in order to grow up toward the cosmos and are a great analogy for our spines and the chakras. Allow this tree grounding to give your conscious or your subconscious mind information about the planet; in other words, the tree has an active and receptive quality. The tree initiates our energetic and conscious relationship with the planet.

When connected, the planet happily accepts and recycles our worries, concerns, stressors, and life challenges. The planet will happily tell you what is up with her. When you are in touch with the planet, jet lag decreases as you tune into shifts in planetary vibration. Your unconscious mind will guide you to a safe place during tumultuous weather, hurricanes and tornados, or earthquakes. The key is to remain calm and centered, which is extremely challenging in times of emergency.

. . . .

••• strawberry affinity tonic •••

Many parents swear by the ability of a delicious smoothie to deliver the much-needed daily requirements of fruits and veggies to children who are picky eaters. This sweet smoothie delivers the power of strawberries, the energetic divine properties of rose water, and the often forgotten benefits of coconut milk.

- ¾ cup strawberries
- 2 tablespoons rose water (see recipe, page 55)
- ¼ cup coconut milk
- 1–2 tablespoons agave nectar for sweetening

Place in a blender, blend, and serve.

... children's banana sorghum shake ...

Yogurt, a superfood, provides beneficial flora for children's intestinal tracts, and aids in overall health of the immune system. This recipe allows you to sweeten the yogurt yourself and avoid excess processed sugar. Sorghum, originally from Africa, is extremely high in much needed minerals for children, including iron and calcium, and used to be prescribed by doctors as a vitamin supplement before there were vitamin pills. (Flax oil supports brain development, critical for young minds.)

- ½ cup unsweetened yogurt (nondairy version use 1¼ cups almond, soy, or rice milk instead of yogurt and water)
- ¾–1 cup water
- 1 banana or any available fruit
- 1–2 tablespoons sorghum
- 1 tablespoon flaxseed oil

Place ingredients in a blender and blend at high speed for 1–2 minutes. A smoothie with lots of vitamins, iron, essential fatty acids, and protein, derived from whole food that even picky eaters will enjoy!

CHAPTER 13

make your own chakra tonics

mAKING YOUR OWN tonics, teas, and elixirs can be simple. I am not a chef; I am a busy mother, partner, yoga teacher, and writer. I developed many of the recipes in this book, using my knowledge of the chakras and accessing my intuition. Using a blender, a juicer, and a teapot, you can come up with your own spontaneous and simple tea, smoothie, and juice recipes.

To attune your elixirs to your energetic needs, cultivate a relationship and understanding of the properties of your ingredients. Look for fresh, seasonal ingredients in the garden, on the farm, at the farmers market, at the health food store, in the plant nursery, or the botanical gardens. If you are new to accessing your intuition and want to start simple, rely at first on your senses; touch, taste, and feel fresh fruits and vegetables. This is the organoleptic approach. Look at ingredients in terms of simple attributes like color.

Even nutritionists recommend eating a wide range of colorful fruits and vegetables. Color contains vibrations and energetic frequencies. On the deepest and most powerful level, plants and foods have spirits. Try to connect as deeply as possible. And this does not mean understanding scientifically what is supposed to be good for you. It is always important to see a physician or health care professional in cases of acute symptoms or illness. Many health conditions may have developed over time and the possibility exists that through eating and drinking more intuitively we will remain in better health.

chakra colors

Root Chakra: Red
Sacral Chakra: Orange
Belly Chakra: Yellow
Heart Chakra: Green
Throat Chakra: Blue
Brow Chakra: Purple
Crown Chakra: White/Ultra Violet/Gold

Before the advent of science, people lived closer to nature and understood their spiritual connection to all living things. There were no scientific studies, wellness magazines, or nutrition websites that told us how to eat or drink. If you live in a rural area, then you may have a greater understanding of the healing power of nature. But there are many ways to connect to plants in a densely populated area. Connecting to the natural world around you will assist you in finding plants and foods that will elevate your spiritual vibration. To find medicinal and culinary herbs, go on plant walks with herbalists, go foraging for wild foliage with horticulturists, or buy a guide to plants in your region.

On a deeper level, develop skills of meditative observation of vegetation. The simplest launch point for our intuition about plants and healing foods is the doctrine of signatures. This is an ancient spiritual concept understood by people around the globe who live close to nature, including, the Aborigines, Native Americans, and even the people of the Appalachian region. It was first written about in Western texts in the writings of a Swiss physician named Hohenheim in the sixteenth century. This idea of looking at the physical characteristics in a plant to discover pharmaceutical value was then further explicated in the early seventeenth century by a German shoemaker, Jacob Boehme, who had a mystic vision regarding the relationship between what he called God and man. He wrote something called *The Signature of All Things,* which conveyed his spiritual philosophy and interestingly was used soon after for its medical applications. The doctrine of signatures is used today in homeopathy, flower-essence treatment, and herbal remedies. It postulates that by observing plants distinguishing characteristics—the color and shape of its flowers, where and how it grows—its spiritual and medicinal properties may be discerned. Shamans delve deeply into the spirit world of plants, in a place beyond the physical senses, where they often clairvoyantly see the spirit of the plants. This highly experiential form of medicine is sometimes hard for Westerners to grasp. Some recommended books on the subject of the spirit of plants are *Plant Spirit Medicine* by Eliot Cowan and *Jungle Medicine* by Connie Grauds, and *The Secret Life of Plants* by Peter Tompkins and Christopher Bird.

Another important concept in making your own healing tonics is to use local, seasonal ingredients. Physical travel and the transport of fruits and vegetables is fast and convenient in modern society. We can enjoy the healing antioxidant power and high levels of vitamin C in kiwis shipped from New Zealand to stave off a winter cold. Supermarkets fool our minds but not our bodies. According to Eliot Cowan, in his book *Plant Spirit Medicine*, British acupuncturist Dr. Worsley shows that herbs that grow in your area have 1,000 times the power of those that do not. There is a spiritual reason you are living where you live. If you have traveled to different countries or even different areas of the United States, you understand that the energy of the earth and culture changes with geography. Unless you are ready to pick up and move because you no longer feel bonded to the area in which you live, you will more likely be healed by eating the plants, edible fruits, and vegetables that reflect the energy of the environment in which they were grown.

There is a huge interest at the moment in learning about and cultivating native plants, which I believe reflects a growing interest in restoring the earth to its natural balance. Not all native plants are medicinal, but many are. There are numerous organizations that can help you learn about native plants in your area. An excellent website to reference is *www.plantnative.org*, or search on your state or region's name and "native plants" and there will likely be a link to your state's native plant organization. Eliot Cowan reminds us that plants love to travel, so the rule of thumb in native plants is to determine whether or not the plant thrives in your local environment.

If you live in an urban area, I urge you to go to a farmers market once a week or once a month. You will see that what is grown locally is very different than what is available in supermarkets. It is a great way to sample new fruits, vegetables, and herbs, and find the freshest, vital, locally grown ingredients for your drinks. Vendors are usually brimming with energy about their food and will often give you ideas and recipes on the spot. Many farmers offer newsletters or boxes of their produce to be sent directly to your home or office. Develop your security in the form of your intuition and enjoy making your own delicious fresh elixirs.

CHAPTER 14

chakra rituals and meditations

a RITUAL IS A SERIES of actions, behaviors, and thoughts enacted with a specific intention. Athletes who perform game-day rituals report feeling more confident and prepared for the heightened challenges of competition. Rituals can enhance performance in daily life too. They direct attention toward positive outcomes and away from negative thoughts, such as worry and doubt. Rituals can help us feel in control even when there are many things out of our control.

The following Chakra Rituals include instructions for actions, reflections, and meditations that will help you to free your chakras and enable life force energy to flow more freely through your body. For some, life force energy seems abstract. If this sounds like you, think about how you feel when you are well rested, relaxed, and present. That's how it feels to have balanced, open chakras and life force flowing through you.

When performed with sacred intentions, the Chakra Rituals will help you to release the past and become more engaged in the present. Chakras can be blocked by negative thoughts and feelings like anxiety, sadness, or upset, and by physical, emotional, and psychological trauma. The Chakra Rituals reduce or eliminate these negative feelings and help you stay connected to what you would like to transform or achieve in mind, body, and spirit. Use these rituals to increase spiritual, emotional, and psychological growth, overcome everyday obstacles, and move forward in your own personal journey of evolution.

Discover what **Chakra Rituals and Meditations** would be best for you by answering the questions on page 71.

root chakra ritual

This ritual is best done outdoors near a tree. Sit on the ground or in a chair, close your eyes, and connect to the feeling and resonance of the earth. Imagine that resonance is a color. Envision little portals or vacuums in the arches of your feet opening up and pulling in the color that represents the earth. Draw the color up into your body through your feet and legs. Allow it to rise through your spine. Let it move down your shoulders, into your arms, and pour out of the center of your hands and fingers. Let some of the earth resonance move up through your legs and spill back into the earth, washing out any disconnection to the earth that might be in your root center at the base of your spine. Observe the color rising through your spine to the top of your head and see it spraying out. As it fountains out of your crown center, visualize it clearing the aura around your body of negative energy. Do this visualization for about three minutes. Finally, hold your tonic in your hands and imagine the earth chi flowing, moving from your hands into your cup or glass, cleansing and grounding your elixir. Do this for about thirty seconds to a minute, then drink and enjoy. Celebrate becoming a living, breathing fountain of earth chi.

Bonus ritual tip: Before starting the Root Chakra Ritual, activate your sense of smell, which is connected to the root chakra. Dab some vetiver, sandalwood, frankincense, or cedarwood essential oil behind your ears or on your wrists.

sacral chakra session

This ritual is best experienced with a watery elixir like tea or juice. You will also need something to taste, such as fresh or dried fruit: peach, orange, apple, dried mango, raisins, etc. Have a pen and journal ready. Hold your glass of tea or tonic in your hands. Observe its liquid quality, then spin the container and observe the movement and flow. What does the elemental property of water mean to you? Think of how you flow through life. Do you sometimes freeze up, or do you allow challenges and triggers to move through you like you are water? Do you take time to ride the choppy waves of life, or do you let them slap you in the face? Set the intention that you will release any blockages to the sacral center. What triggers you and causes you to get defensive, upset, or angry? There is no need to blame yourself; this is an exploration of your energy and to discern how to flow. We cannot control other people or many circumstances. This chakra helps us find a way to be honest, yet calm, when we are triggered. Imagine a color, possibly a shade of blue (the color of water) or orange (the traditional color of this chakra). Let this color flow through the top of your head and wash through all of your chakras, especially the sacral center. The chakras are connected, just like water. The sacral chakra helps us to react internally, and using that information wisely helps us to move forward. We often need self-empathy and love to move ahead and onward. Now take your fruit, symbolizing sweetness and sensuality. When in season, a peach would be the finest choice for this ritual. Take the fruit and look at it; anticipate its flavor. Take a small piece of fruit and place it in your mouth. Do not chew at first. Notice its texture and preliminary flavor. Then chew very slowly, savoring the flavor, texture, and anything else you notice. Chew at least twenty-six times. Finally swallow. Then sit and eat the rest of your fruit and drink your Chakra Tonic. Journal on anything you learned about yourself in this ritual.

belly center morning ritual

This morning practice was inspired by my parents who read a print newspaper daily. For the purposes of this ritual, imagine you are holding a newspaper. This ritual is best done in the morning to awaken energy and to get morning light to stimulate your internal energetic clock that governs your circadian rhythms.

Go outside where there is natural light before ten o'clock in your time zone. Stand and think about embracing the day. What does that mean to you? Do you already feel drained, or do you feel invigorated by your schedule? Next, imagine you are picking up a newspaper off the ground. Bend down and pick up the imaginary newspaper. Hold it over your head and stretch upward. Repeat this bending and lifting gesture at least five times. This stretch wakes your circulatory system (energy). Now pause and hold the imaginary newspaper near your belly, which symbolically is your reservoir of chi. Imagine the news contains all the information you need to remain present and alert. All you need to do is show up. Then, take the invisible newspaper to your heart and hold it there. Take in only the "news" that uplifts you and matches your purpose. Leave any other world or unsolved problems for others who are called to solve these problems. The belly center aligns us with our purpose and passion. Filter out anything that does not align with your spiritual purpose. This ritual helps you to stay energized and keeps you connected to your purpose and power. It can help restore faith in your spiritual path, because we are so often drained by things we have no control over. Let everything else go with the faith that there are healthy, balanced humans who will take care of the problems that you cannot in this moment. The belly center governs the sense of sight, so complete the ritual by honoring that sense. Look around you, observing the morning light and what you see.

Bonus ritual tip: Bounce on your heels and shake out your wrists, arms, and legs one at a time. Do this for thirty seconds and up to two minutes. Follow this by a walk. If you don't have time for a walk, march in place, touching the opposite arm to leg to balance the two hemispheres of the brain.

Offer a toast to your vitality as you drink your Chakra Tonic outside in the morning light.

anahata arrival

Anahata means "unstruck." This ritual can be done sitting or standing. Begin by tapping or gently striking your sternum with your pointer, middle, and ring fingers of your right or left hand. As you tap on your heart center, repeat the following heart-based affirmations.

- ✦ I love myself unconditionally.
- ✦ I love my true nature.
- ✦ I forgive myself.

- ✦ I am divine.
- ✦ Love is inside me and guiding my actions.
- ✦ I made a mistake, how human of me.
- ✦ I am grateful for _____(name three to five things)
- ✦ I am open to receiving love from those I choose to receive love from.

Tap and speak the affirmations for five to ten minutes, repeating your favorite phrases. Release any feelings of disconnection from your heart, and connect to a sense of self-love. To close this ritual, shut your eyes and visualize your heart as a flower of your choice. Traditionally the heart chakra is represented by a lotus flower. Now look at it and ask yourself:

- ✦ How open is your flower?
- ✦ Is it a bud, fully in bloom, or beginning to wither?
- ✦ What does your heart need to blossom?

See an image or sense what your heart center needs. Your needs count and your heart has a gauge that cannot be ignored. Contemplate how to meet your needs in a healthy way, since your heart's needs are essential. Complete this ritual with a joyful toast to yourself! Sip your tea or tonic while you extend loving kindness towards yourself.

visiting with vishuddha

After preparing your Chakra Tonic, find a song or chant to sing for five minutes. You may want to recite the Bija mantras, "Lam Yam, Ram, Ham, Vram, Om." More information on the Bija mantras can be found on page 37. There are many YouTube videos that loop the Bija mantras that you can chant to. Karaoke is a great throat center balancing activity. Notice if you love your voice or if you feel self-conscious, or if you do not like or sometimes even loathe the sound of your voice. The more you sing, chant, and listen, the more you will hear and love your voice. Close the ritual with the opposite of sound—silence—while you visualize the color blue. Close your eyes and visualize yourself surrounded by a sky-blue bubble. Breathe in blue and breathe out anything blocking that color or your expression. Do this for three to five minutes.

Bonus ritual tip: Do this ritual early in the morning and drink your tonic outside while listening to birdsong.

ajna activation

Do this candlelit ritual at night with a tea; the Cloud 9 Astral Travel Tea (page 155) would be a good choice. The traditional yoga practice of Trataka cleanses and purifies the mind. It promotes intuition and increases the strength of our visioning by activating the brow center. This inner knowingness is called the third eye, because we may see something unsaid or unknown. (This is different than a gut intuition or hearing an inaudible "voice.") According to the Vedic texts and Hatha Yoga Pradipika, to practice Trataka, stare at a flickering lit candle and concentrate on the flame. Sometimes you may see an image in your mind's eye. Even if you don't see anything, the candle gazing traditionally cleanses the intuitive third eye. Meditate on the flame, allowing your mind to clear and release. Allow the flame's dance to sense your connection to light and its movement. Look at the candle without blinking until your eyes tear up. Then close your eyes and visualize the flame for one to three minutes. You may want to sip your tea during Trataka or wait until you have finished the ritual. Do this ritual at night just before bed for sound sleep.

cosmic crown activation

This ritual goes well with a light tea and is best done early in the morning or just before bed. The crown center is about zooming out and seeing yourself as a part of a greater whole. The crown center connects us with the highest intelligence, vastness of the universe, and the unity of all people, animals, places, cultures, and the planet. It helps you to feel connected to all beings, stars, and galaxies. From your crown center, you see the good in all things, and you can easily pray for someone in need. Never force yourself to feel or be connected to the divine or you will cause a spiritual bypass and lose your opportunity for growth and evolution. Spiritual bypass is a concept first expressed by Buddhist teacher and psychologist John Welwood to describe spiritual practitioners who used spiritual concepts or practices to avoid or bypass their own pain. Like a drug, a practice of spiritual bypass causes us to avoid processing pain and trauma and remain stunted or stalled in our evolutionary growth.

Write down or think of three things you are grateful for. Drink your tea from the feeling of gratitude, forgiveness, and reverence. These feelings will be challenged when we go through trauma, challenges, or great difficulty, but these challenges can help us more deeply connect to divine source. It is human to not be able to access this chakra. When you find yourself feeling disconnected from divine source, visualize God or the highest energy of the universe as a color. Meditate on this color and imagine letting it pour into the crown of your head and into every cell of your body. When you are filled with this color, continue to focus on appreciation and write down a minimum of three things that you feel immense gratitude for. Keep this list handy and read it at night before bed or in the morning when you wake up.

APPENDIX
directory of contributors

FOR THE LAST 10 YEARS, JUICEY LUCY'S has been a pioneering organic vegetarian kosher cafe, tucked in between ubiquitous pizza and pasta joints in the celebrated North Beach neighborhood of San Francisco at 703 Columbus Avenue at Filbert. Accolades from *Gourmet* magazine, voted best juice bar in San Francisco by SF Weekly readers, *Super Smoothies* authors and sisters Mary Corpening Barber and Sara Corpening Whiteford, and San Francisco food guru Patricia Unterman are a result of the restaurant's creative menu of seasonal, local ingredients. Sit down as Lisa Bach personally alchemizes your meal from a rainbow of fresh-picked produce that seems to grow from right behind the counter. Her juices are pure sattva, like their mantra "Juice and food that takes you up and never lets you down." Website: *www.juiceylucys.com,* 415-786-1285.

KAMI MCBRIDE is an herbalist, healer and women's health advocate, and director of Living Awareness Institute. Her parents brought her up with plenty of experience in wild nature, which she hopes to pass on to future generations. She has studied with many of the luminaries of the herbal and metaphysical world, including Vicki Noble, Dr. Vasant Lad, Michael Moore, and Candace Cantin. Kami contributed recipes in chapters 4 and 5. She is also the author of *The Herbal Kitchen*. She can be contacted at *www.livingawareness.com*.

Christie McClelland is director of the Gayatri Institute, which offers classes and an eight-week well-being cleanse, where participants cleanse the body in a supportive group with the help of a diverse board of integrative health care professionals. Christie has been meditating since the age of nine and has studied many healing modalities, including yoga and massage. *www.gayatri.elly.org*.

Caitlin Phillips is a flower essence and gem elixir specialist and contributed a list of gem elixirs for the chakras. She has studied flower and gem essences in Australia and Bali. She studied with and did private consultations at the world's only exclusive flower essence store, Audrey's Good Vibrations in Venice Beach, California. She gives spiritual counseling and aura and chakra readings and can be reached at *caitlinpmk@yahoo.com*.

SHAZZIE is a raw-food chef, healthy-living advocate, and author of *Detox Your World*. A glamorous and pure health fanatic, Shazzie is a "mum," a raw-food publicist, chef, writer, and entrepreneur. Her website, *www.detoxyourworld.com*, is a worldwide destination for detox converts.

JAY DEVA KUMAR, M.A., Ph.D. candidate, is a Sanskrit scholar, therapeutic yoga teacher, Ayurvedic consultant, and contributing editor to *Yoga Journal* magazine. He gave an interview about the sacred language of Sanskrit and its relationship to the chakras. He can be contacted at 415-641-8300 or through his website *www.drjaykumar.com*. He has created an accessible and down-to-earth guide to Sanskrit that comes with a CD. It's called *The Sacred Language of Yoga: A Sanskrit Guide to the Philosophy, Mantras, and Vocabulary in the Yoga Tradition*. Because written text is limited in conveying the complex pronunciations of Sanskrit, this guide is highly recommended for further study of mantras and chakras.

about the author

Elise Marie Collins is a yoga teacher, writer, and spiritual counselor. A graduate of the Berkeley Psychic Institute and University of California, Berkeley, she has written for *Yoga Journal* and other alternative health magazines, and was the Body and Soul columnist for *Psychic Reader*. Her latest book, *Super Ager: You Can Look Younger, Have More Energy, a Better Memory, and Live a Long and Healthy Life*, published in 2018, is an Amazon bestseller. Her other book is *An A-Z Guide to Healing Foods: A Shopper's Reference*. Find out more about her offerings at www.elisemariecollins.com.

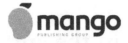

Mango Publishing, established in 2014, publishes an eclectic list of books by diverse authors—both new and established voices—on topics ranging from business, personal growth, women's empowerment, LGBTQ studies, health, and spirituality to history, popular culture, time management, decluttering, lifestyle, mental wellness, aging, and sustainable living. We were recently named 2019 and 2020's #1 fastest-growing independent publisher by *Publishers Weekly*. Our success is driven by our main goal, which is to publish high-quality books that will entertain readers as well as make a positive difference in their lives.

Our readers are our most important resource; we value your input, suggestions, and ideas. We'd love to hear from you— after all, we are publishing books for you!

Please stay in touch with us and follow us at:
Facebook: Mango Publishing
Twitter: @MangoPublishing
Instagram: @MangoPublishig
LinkedIn: Mango Publishing
Pinterest: Mango Publishing
Newsletter: mangopublishinggroup.com/newsletter

Join us on Mango's journey to reinvent publishing, one book at a time.

CPSIA information can be obtained
at www.ICGtesting.com
Printed in the USA
LVHW041106020622
720263LV00004B/271